Parkinson's Disease

My Brain This Time

By Elliot Essman

Copyright © Elliot Essman 2021
www.elliotessman.com

Table of Contents

Preface

Two men speak through the centuries

Stephen Hopkins, former governor of Rhode Island, waited with the other delegates to sign the document, knowing, as did all assembled, that he could in effect be signing his own death warrant. The fifty-six men gathered in Philadelphia that summer came from all walks of life: lawyers, farmers, a printer, a brewer, a cobbler. We tend to think of revolutionaries as wild-eyed people wielding rifles, shouting slogans. These men wielded quill pens, in a battle that to them centered on thirteen hundred words: the Declaration of American Independence. Hopkins had to wait for the Massachusetts men to sign: Samuel Adams, his cousin John Adams, Robert Treat Paine and Elbridge Gerry. The Rhode Island delegation, just two men, then took their turn. William Ellery of Newport deferred to Hopkins, who walked only with difficulty. Hopkins approached the table tentatively, his hands shaking uncontrollably, not from the gravity of the moment, not from fear of a British noose, but from an ailment people at that time called the "shaking palsy," what we now call Parkinson's disease. Hopkins took up the quill with his right hand and steadied the hand with his left. If you look at a good image of the Declaration, so familiar to us, you can make out his signature today in the right-most column of names, about halfway down, using extra space for all the effort it took, threatening in its inelegance to slide off the edge of the parchment.

"My hand trembles," Hopkins told the others as he signed, "but my heart does not."

The words are stirring, but from the perspective of what we know of history now, I would like to put it a different way: "One man trembled, but the entire world shook."

The year was, as we know, 1776. Across the Atlantic in England, James Parkinson was twenty-one years old, preparing to enter his father's apothecary and medical practice in Hoxton, a part of the East End of London. Within a few years, Parkinson was authorized to practice surgery, but he was also a political man. With American independence, many people in England, Parkinson included, began to agitate for a fairer system of parliamentary election and wider suffrage. The French revolution of 1789 only emboldened these political critics, whose key inspiration became Thomas Paine's 1791 book *Rights of Man*. Writing anonymously under the name of "Old Hubert," Parkinson published more than twenty political pamphlets calling for radical social reforms. The anonymity was necessary. Parkinson risked prosecution, prison, or even transportation to the penal colony in Australia for these activities, the fate of a number of his associates. The repression in Britain became particularly aggressive after the French revolution descended into the terror and mass murder of 1793-94. Parkinson managed to skate through this difficult period, stepping back from politics when Napoleon took over in France and became an external threat to the British nation. Through all this, his medical practice in Hoxton flourished.

With the coming of the 19th century, Parkinson became something of the Doctor Oz of his day, publishing the guides *Medical Admonitions to Families* in 1801, *The Villager's Friend and Physician* in 1804, and *Dangerous Sports* in 1808 (in which he counseled young people to wear the equivalent of a helmet while doing rough and tumble activities). His medical research led to groundbreaking investigations of gout (which plagued him) and appendicitis. Always socially concerned, he agitated for public health programs (including vaccination for smallpox) and legal protection for the mentally ill, whom he treated for over twenty-five years at the infamous Hoxton "madhouse." Beyond medicine, the ever-inquisitive Parkinson did comprehensive studies of geology and paleontology. He was a pioneer in the identification of fossils, and amassed the largest fossil collection in Britain. His *Organic Remains of a Former World* (1804-1811) became the foremost reference work on paleontology for the first half of the nineteenth century. He also found time to turn out a popular chemistry handbook that went through four editions between 1800 and 1807.

Parkinson was already over sixty when he published his comprehensive study of what he called "paralysis agitans" in 1817, *An Essay on the Shaking Palsy*, which he defined as:

> "Involuntary tremulous motion, with lessened muscular power…with a propensity to bend the trunk forwards…the senses and intellects being uninjured."

The essay established the disease as a recognized medical condition. Parkinson died in 1824. It would be another half century before pioneering French neurologist Jean-Martin Charcot gave the condition the name "Parkinson's disease." It was only in the mid-twentieth century that the drug Levodopa became available to allay some of the symptoms. The disease remains difficult to diagnose, yet there comes a time when if you have Parkinson's disease you know it.

I have it and I know it.

James Parkinson was a remarkable man, worth
commemorating for so much more than the disease that
bears his name, but Stephen Hopkins (1707-1785) was also
multi-dimensional. Hopkins served as governor of Rhode
Island for nine terms, and Chief Justice of the Rhode Island
Supreme Court. A close friend of Benjamin Franklin,
Hopkins in 1764 published an article entitled "The Rights
of the Colonies Examined," calling for unification of the
colonies as one nation. The second oldest signer (after
Franklin), Hopkins came to Philadelphia the most
unwavering of patriots. He was a man of exceptional
learning, a skilled surveyor and astronomer—he served as
part of the American contingent that recorded the "transit
of Venus" across the sun in 1769, part of an international
effort that helped gauge the distance between the sun and
the planets. He was also a successful merchant,
entrepreneur, newspaper publisher, and one of the earliest
proponents of paper currency (which some of us still use
today). The nature of these writings compels me to use
Parkinson's name on nearly every page, but before I do
that, I want to give Stephen Hopkins a parting homage, and
take his choice Philadelphia words as my own.

My hand also trembles, but my heart does not.

When the earth trembles and shakes, fruit falls from the trees

Introduction

I write these words to get to the bottom of it all.

As a trained professional in the business of alcoholic beverages, I have long lived with a poignant bit of irony. Strong drink rarely makes me drunk, or even tipsy. Maybe it is my focus on quality—I do not drink swill—maybe just something in my blood, or perhaps it is simply insufficient volume. You might jump to the conclusion that my inability to inebriate myself is some kind of asset, a valuable tool if I am, say, negotiating over a business lunch. This might come into play if I did not live the solitary life of the writer. Sometimes I get so wound up that I need the release of drunkenness, but all I get is a pleasant gustatory experience: a fine wine on my nose and palate, the solace of a single malt scotch, a bit of *fuego* from a Tequila or Mezcal. Even here, I need to accept the reality that my senses of taste and smell have been both compromised by Parkinson's.

Now that I have Parkinson's disease, I teeter and totter and might as well be drunk as a skunk much of the time, *except* when I actually drink. I imagine being stopped at a police sobriety check, showing a zero level of alcohol on the breathalyzer and yet proving unable to walk a straight line—big judgment issue for the cop. I drink most evenings, long after I have put my car to bed. During the day, far from a bottle, I lurch down the street. I attract stares. Do I care? Yes, I do, but then I do not. I have an ailment, it does not go away, and yet, though it is a part of my life, it is not the whole story. I write these words to get to the bottom of it all, in the same sense that I would gradually get to the bottom of a bottle of wine, upending the thing to coax out the final precious drops.

Parkinson's disease is a progressive disorder of the nervous system that affects movement. The most likely cause is an inability of the brain to generate a substance called dopamine, which regulates muscular movement. As with any disease or health issue, hundreds of books and guides for patients and families are available—I have greatly profited from several good ones—but this is a different kind of book, a personal memoir, by a writer whose field of expertise is otherwise wine and spirits. However introspective or philosophical I might be about Parkinson's (I majored in philosophy at a Jesuit university), I face the unalterable fact that I have the disease and undergo treatment for it, taking medications several times a day, watching my diet, exercising, taking on the thing one day at a time. I suffer from weakness, trembling and pain on my left side, fatigue, breathing issues, diminished senses of taste and smell, and difficulty balancing myself. I not only feel that I am liable to fall down, but also experience a sensation of floating up into the stratosphere. Now, with Parkinson's, I feel at least slightly drunk more often than not.

The disease is still very new for me, but one thing is already clear: after any type of activity, I need to stand back from the experience, process it, recover from it, in both body and mind. That is the gist: acting, even thinking, in discrete stages instead of fluidly sliding through life. The multitasking so integral to modern life is virtually impossible. To consume a piece of fruit, I must coax it out of the produce bag (the bag fights me on this), remove the stick-on label, wash the fruit, find a surface, knife off chunks, open the trash, let gravity take care of the pit or core, close the trash—the gravity step alone is without effort. With Parkinson's, no activity is seamless: I get my left foot into a shoe, adjust my heel, tie the shoe, do the same for the right foot, and thank god there are only the

pair! I must plan ordinary events. The smallest task forces
me to strategize—how am I going to get this one done?

Parkinson's disease is often hard to spot, and hence not
easy to diagnose. You cannot reach a definitive diagnosis
with a blood test or an MRI. If you have a basket of typical
Parkinson's symptoms, you *might* have the disease. If
medication works to alleviate some or most of the
symptoms, you *probably* have the disease. This is my case,
although I have two additional markers for the disease: I
tested positive for the *leucine-rich repeat kinase 2 (LRRK2)*
gene, prevalent in people of Ashkenazi Jewish descent, and
had a Dopamine Transmission (DaT) scan, which found a
dopamine transmission deficiency. I am now at a level of
equilibrium, but this has taken a full four years—forty-
eight months—from my first symptoms. These happen to
coincide with four calendar years—the first symptoms were
a grim January gift, and as I write this it is only a few
weeks until Santa comes and brings me—well, why not full
and complete health?

I ought to stress here that when I talk about "symptoms," I
refer only to those severe enough to show on my radar. It is
sadly common for people with Parkinson's to suffer from a
range of symptoms long before they realize they might
have a neurological problem: sleep issues, anxiety,
dizziness, constipation, urinary annoyances, difficulty
breathing, odd aches and pains, muscle pulsations, and the
most insidious villain of them all, unexplained fatigue. Like
many, I likely had dopamine deficiency issues long before
the chronology that follows. Part of current research into
Parkinson's involves identifying "bio-markers," substances
in saliva, blood or cerebrospinal fluid that could
conceivably flag the disease earlier. For precisely this
purpose, I am presently a volunteer test subject for the
Parkinson's Progression Markers Initiative (PPMI)

sponsored by the Michael J. Fox Foundation for Parkinson's Research.

Here is a rough chronology.

In **month one**, I began to have disturbing episodes of feeling light-headed and woozy, a feeling of depersonalization, of looking down on myself from the ceiling, a sensation of lack of control, combined with an extremely nervous feeling. I saw no physician for this, figuring it was all my old pal, anxiety (which I will write about later, at length). My prescription for myself—and it was a good one—single malt Scotch. I believe at this time I was slowly working through a bottle of Oban. In thinking back on it, I can taste heather, some warm spice, honeysuckle and a light touch of violet, no peat. The finish was long, but night took its toll, and in a few days I got the feeling again. Months then fluttered off the calendar with no incident at all.

A pulsating pain in my left calf had been annoying me for a while, but since my hobby was hiking up mountains (in Albuquerque, New Mexico), I decided the pain and discomfort was just something I had to accept as the overhead of my passion. Then came **month seven**, when I felt the entire left side of my body collapse in weakness, arm and hand included. My first fear was a stroke or heart event, but fourteen hours in the local emergency room ruled these out. None of the medical personnel who examined me thought to suggest that I might have a neurologic problem. Their verdict was "musculoskeletal pain." I asked, "what about the weakness in my arm," but I got the reply, "Let's concentrate on the leg."

I was sick, lonely, and a bit depressed. I also had great difficulty breathing because of the seasonal tree allergies (if it isn't juniper, it is mountain sage). I packed up and moved from Albuquerque back to my origin in New York, to be closer to my family.

In **month ten**, after a spinal MRI, I learned that I had an orthopedic problem, a bulging disk in my lower spine that they said was responsible for the pains in my left leg. In **months eleven and twelve**, I had epidural pain treatments—they accomplished nothing. I asked both the orthopedist and the pain doctor about the achiness and weakness in my arm and hand, and again was told, "let us first fix the leg."

Around **month eleven**, I began to think I had movement issues. Taking keys out of my pocket was becoming a less-than-automatic event, as was getting dressed, undressed, or opening an envelope. I often felt frozen, unable to move. My voice, once loud, became uncharacteristically soft. I had trouble breathing. My regular doctor was able to help with the breathing, but he could not make the jump to the possibility of Parkinson's—a trained Parkinson's specialist could have zeroed in on it with a five-minute examination. I did not think of it. To me Parkinson's involved involuntary shaking and little else. I did not even look it up on the Internet. I got through my days with painkillers and through my nights with sleeping aids.

My next step was physical therapy. I got a prescription for this from my regular doctor, which mentioned that I was having difficulty with my leg. I went for twenty sessions in **months thirteen and fourteen**. A team of brutal sadists worked my legs hard. "I also have issues with my left hand and arm," I protested, but to no avail. My left arm twitched. My three leftmost fingers rebelled against any form of keyboard work, either at my computer or on my piano.

After using all the physical therapy sessions that my insurance allowed, I began to believe that I had a neurological problem. In **month sixteen** I saw **Neurologist One** (out of three). After several MRIs and a lumbar punch fluoroscopy, she diagnosed me with multiple sclerosis. She prescribed the drug Copaxone, which I needed to inject every day. I followed a diet specifically designed for MS, travelling to Whole Foods Market at least once a week to buy my line-caught salmon. Broccoli was heavily involved, and so too kale, in every form, raw, cooked, dried, chips—I stuffed it in until I could hardly breathe. The very word kale makes me cringe now! Kale, like all panaceas, is evil. Down with kale!

In **month twenty-three**, I visited an MS specialist to get a second opinion. **Neurologist Two** put me through new MRIs, told me I had Parkinson's disease and not MS, questioning the basic competence of Neurologist One. She took me off the Copaxone and started me on Carbidopa-Levodopa at the end of **month twenty-five**, more than two years into the sequence (and after more than eight months of useless Copaxone injections). Some months later, I got around to making an appointment with a Parkinson's specialist. I had to wait four months for the appointment, which finally occurred in **month thirty-four**. **Neurologist Three** started by giving me some legal advice. "You can sue her," he said of Neurologist One. "I have never seen such negligence." I followed through on the legal line immediately. (I also have a law degree from the same Jesuit university in which I majored in philosophy.) I went through extensive interviews with two malpractice law firms, more than an hour of questions in both instances, but neither law firm smelled enough money to want to get involved.

After Neurologist Three cooled down from his diatribe over the negligence of Neurologist One, he also had choice words for Neurologist Two. "She made the correct diagnosis," he told me, "You do have Parkinson's disease, but she has been under-dosing you." He instructed me to take a month to gradually double my dosage of Carbidopa-Levodopa, and then, in **month thirty-five**, add a second drug, Selegiline. I followed his instructions, which required dosing myself three times a day, carefully counting and splitting pills as I slowly doubled the dose.

At about the same time as my first session with Neurologist Three, I received an e-mail from a Milanese public relations firm, inviting me to fly over to northern Italy for several days to review an obscure Piemontese red wine called Ruchè di Castagnole Monferrato. Even though I was devoid of energy, I agreed to go. (You just don't turn down a free trip to Italy.) By the time I flew, in **month thirty-six**, December, I was a week or ten days into the Selegiline. I got to Milan early in the morning. A driver brought me to my hotel. About five pm that evening, Massimo, a local winemaker, and his English-speaking niece Allesandra picked me up. They took me to their winery and cellar, we tasted several wines, and then they showed me the village. These towns are hilly, as are the vineyards. For some reason I had energy, although I was expecting jetlag to hit me any second. We parked in the village square. They led me on foot up a steep street. The ancient village church stood at the top. I found myself bounding up the steps of that stone church, not even slightly out of breath. I looked back at my hosts, who were probably thinking here is the American showing off his physical prowess—typical. I knew better. I knew it was the new drug, Selegiline, working. I took in the moment, certain I was not the first traveler to have a moment of epiphany in Italy.

I had a long evening ahead of me, primarily at a local restaurant. Winemakers drifted in to join the group all evening. I tasted every possible permutation of Ruchè di Castagnole Monferrato: still, sparkling, dry and sweet. The dishes kept appearing in front of me: antipasti, pastas, polenta, vegetables, mushrooms, meats, risotto, superb cheeses, glorious Piemontese desserts, gelato. I can certainly appreciate fine food and drink, and I did, but possibilities, combined with capabilities, swirled through my brain. One of the Italians remarked on my warm smile, on the glow I was radiating. I said, yes, it was the wine, but it was not the wine, it was the prospect of getting my life back.

After I finished writing and publishing fourteen articles about the Italian wine trip, I began to turn the rough journals I had been keeping into this book about Parkinson's disease. Had the new medication made those jottings irrelevant? I told myself no. They show the full force of despair and hope I felt as I was writing them. They capture the essence of the disease as it collides with the human, this human, and I want to retain their firm, and grim, reality.

I know deep in the background of my brain that the drugs I take like clockwork might one day cease to work. They do not work on all the symptoms all the time. Sometimes I have a bad few hours. I shake and cringe. Other times, entire days fall into the sea. I am well enough so that nobody notices but me, but you are never free of this…thing.

Parkinson's is like driving through a construction zone. The sign the worker holds has two sides: stop, and slow.

The Problem With All Those Bags

Are supermarket produce bags created just to test my endurance?

"Here. Let me help you," a woman trailing kids offers. She sees me struggling with a plastic produce bag. I allow her to slip the wisp of a bag from my straining fingers. I do not see how, but in a snap she has the bag open, engulfed with air, freed of static, ready to accept vegetables or fruit. I look her over. She has been opening bags this way for many decades. These are her grandchildren. The kids want her away from the odd teetering man. I want to tell her I have grandchildren this age, but I only have time for thanks. Our eyes meet a half second. She sees, perhaps, that I have "something." The kids pull her away, but as I sort through the apples, she cocks her head back just to make sure I am all right. She knows I will need more than one bag, but this is all she can do.

Plastic bags—designed for convenience—oh is that so? I dispute this statement. I have Parkinson's disease, with diminished finger dexterity and a compromised ability to coordinate in space. Beyond the Parkinson's, I find myself (last I looked) male. Lacking good point precision abilities, I could never, pre-Parkinson's, open those supermarket produce bags without making a production of it. Now—and I do not care who watches—the process is genuine theater: Act I, Scene I, Scene II, and so forth. It just goes to show that you can uncover drama anywhere.

I realize produce comes from the ground (if you except hydroponics), but I figure why encourage further market grime and hand contact. The bag means that the dirt stops here. Call me paranoid or dirt-phobic if you must, but I am convinced the black rubber roller at the checkout counter is a veritable repository of disease, a pathogenic amalgam of an entire community. Fish and meats leak onto the surface, babes in arms sneeze and slobber. I cringe when I see people placing loose fruits and vegetables on the roller. They plan presumably to wash the produce before they consume it, but who sanitizes their spinach, who cleanses their cantaloupe? You rinse it, you eat it, and you hope it doesn't sicken you. I am all for the concept of hope, but when I purchase fruits and vegetables, I believe the fewer human contact points the better.

The first task in the produce bag saga is finding a dispenser. Once I have zeroed in on a roll of bags, I need to reach into the deepest core of my athleticism to extract a single bag from the roll without blanketing the aisle in a snakelike covering of spent bags.

The bag is only a theoretical bag—it's actually a wafer-thin slab of plastic. It is up to me, not an employee, not the manufacturer, to turn the flat slab into a three-dimensional produce carrier. The battle is always uphill: shake the bag, rub the edges, try to get a fingernail in, scrunch the thing in your fist, take on a helpless look in an attempt to attract female assistance. (Picture Edvard Munch's "The Scream," with the character awash in plastic produce bags.) Somehow, someway, I am going to get a bag off the dispenser and get the top of it slightly opened. I can then take a moment to recover and another few seconds to remember why I wanted the bag in the first place.

If I stick my hand into a slightly opened bag to try to plumb its depth, I could encounter resistance and start to teeter. My technique, still in the process of perfection, involves holding the edge of the bag with my strong right fingers and skating my weak left fingers around the inner rim of the open end of the bag. Ideally this will get the bag open enough to try an exploratory piece of produce. Once the item is safely ensconced in the upper reaches of the bag I then use the satisfying certainty of gravity (it is a law) and shake the bag so the item drops down, opening up the bag for further deposits at the same time. This works best with heavy fruit like avocadoes, peaches and plums, less well with lighter, smaller fruit like apricots.

Getting vegetables into a bag is another matter entirely. Their size brings on a situation in which their rough edges cling to the sides of the bag, necessitating further engineering. A head of broccoli is the most difficult (I eat a great deal of broccoli). Here, gravity loses the battle with friction and I have to finesse the sides of the bag up over the clingy florets on a north, south, east, west basis, truly a triumph, but exhausting. The pre-cut, pre-wrapped broccoli florets are a pricier option to which I often succumb, especially considering the certainty that I will later have trouble getting the broccoli *out* of the bag if I use one, and further difficulty cutting the broccoli into pieces to put into my steamer.

You can see now how I juggle gravity, friction, and the tactile behavior of plastics, showing how much science is actually involved in the produce section (beyond the agriculture). As for the bags, I am going to keep using them. Sanitation is only one issue here. The other is dexterity. Without the bags, I will have to fish out every piece of fruit and bit of vegetable individually out of my larger shopping bag when I bring it all home, and the task seems akin to building one of the pyramids without all those slaves to help. When your brain is on trial every day, you get into the dreary habit of factoring every possible physical transaction into your planning, and you start to minimize those events. Think P-for Parkinson's, P-for Planning.

The Parkinson's-challenged muscles that fail to receive the brain's messages are not restricted to those required to manipulate plastic bags, or pump iron at the gym. The human voice calls upon a subtle array of muscles. If these muscles do not work well, in tandem as they should, a faint rasp is often all you get.

Compromise my voice, and you threaten my being.

What Happened to My Voice?

I just want to scream. I said scream!

"Thank you for the wonderful introduction," I say, taking a scan of my audience. "Out of all the introductions I have ever received this one is the most…how shall I put it…recent."

I get some quality light laughs from this remark. It's undemanding and pleasantly ridiculous. When I used to speak in front of groups, I would use this icebreaker about once a year. You will note my use of the past tense here: *used to* speak. Parkinson's menaces my very voice now.

I first got involved in public speaking when, at age thirty-five, I joined a Toastmasters club. I discovered that unlike many people who fear public speaking, I actually craved an audience. I might be nervous interacting with people on a one-on-one basis, but put me in front of a room full of listeners and I come into my element. Public speaking makes me feel whole and calm, centered and steady. Many people will admit to having an actual fear of public speaking (worse than death, some say!) I did not have time for that. My great fear was (and is) the opposite—the fear of being silenced!

During my early public speaking days, others would often counsel me to speak up and project my voice. It seemed the simplest thing to push air out of my mouth, but the key to vocal volume eluded me for some time. I tried and tried, but it could only come out softly. I kept at it, often visualizing that I had the ability to project my voice. The moment of epiphany came when suddenly I could fill halls with my voice, no microphone required. I competed in and won numerous public speaking contests, both serious and humorous. I took joy in helping others break through barriers in public speaking and actually succeeded in bringing across the skill of vocal projection. It is mainly a question of emotional focus. With my newfound skill, I addressed community groups on social issues. I spoke every chance I got, and encouraged others to do the same. I came into my element as a speaker. I considered my voice to be a chalice, a jewel, my essence.

The voice I treasure now suffers from my Parkinson's disease. French neurologist Jean-Martin Charcot, who coined the term "Parkinson's disease," observed that, "the utterance is slow, jerky, and short of phrase." Shakespeare is on the mark as usual when in his "Seven Ages of Man" from *As You Like It*, in the sixth age, he refers to, "his big manly voice, turning again towards childish treble, pipes and whistles in his sound." Many people with the disease have speech and voice issues, including soft voice, a monotonic way of speaking, hoarseness and breathiness, and difficulty articulating words. I am no exception. The medication has improved my energy levels and ability to coordinate myself physically, but I still have issues with my voice. People often ask me to repeat myself or to clarify something I have said. If I say anything with humorous or metaphorical value, I often fail to get my point across for lack of vocal inflection. My voice sounds reedy and thin. The voice cracks in the middle of words, collapses in the middle of sentences. My own ears, from the inside, often cannot hear the difference.

Just today, I was talking to a friend at the gym. He said he was going to Philadelphia for a flower show. I asked, "Are you in the flower business?" He made me repeat the question twice before it registered (no, he simply liked flowers). Five minutes later, I was picking up a prescription at the pharmacy. "I don't need a bag," I volunteered. The drugs come in a small paper bag, to which instructions are stapled. The clerk put the paper bag of drugs into a plastic bag. "I don't need a bag," I repeated, a little more loudly, tapping the gym bag slung over my shoulder. She heard me, and removed the bag from the bag. I realized she hadn't registered any speech from me at all when I had made my first statement. My voice seemed perfectly loud from the inside. It made me wonder—do I need to shout?

There are several theories as to what causes the loss of vocal ability for the Parkinson's patient. The less than adequate muscle motivation that affects my arms and legs may also affect the muscles that regulate speech. There is also the question of reduced sensory processing: my brain forms speech, but I have lost the sensory ability to gauge how loudly and accurately the speech is coming out. My brain also has lost some of its ability to cue my voice to adequate loudness. As with other activities, what used to be automatic now requires a volitional decision. In normal conversation, I need to push my voice out as if I were addressing a group: formally, with planning, with deliberation and care, otherwise others will not understand what I am trying to say. I get feedback from others and know they have trouble registering my feeble efforts. My voice was once my joy, and now it is but another in a long line of Parkinson's frustrations.

The First Amendment to the United States Constitution mandates that "Congress shall make no law…abridging the freedom of speech." This restriction also applies to the individual states and all their legal subdivisions: counties, towns, villages, school boards, conservation districts, water and sewage authorities—what have you. The government may not abridge your freedom of speech, but your own fears can stifle that freedom very nicely. It happened to me. Parkinson's was not the first force to threaten me with silence. I first began to struggle with this concept when I was only a few years old. In the face of a stampede, I was but a blade of grass. My father was a narcissistic loudmouth. The steam of talk had no end—in fact, it had no beginning—it was constant and continual. The man was always right, as a first principle, which meant that all other opinions and points of view were consequentially wrong. Of course, I did not understand what he was spewing about when I was two, but the volume, quantity and tone of the words had their inhibitory effect.

I did not speak a word until I was three. There did not seem to be much point. Nothing was done for me, no treatment suggested. Did I have a physical problem with my brain, or was my silence strictly of emotional or psychological origin? The answer is lost. Today, if the child does not speak on cue within a week of the developmental stage at which he is "supposed" to speak, the parents will worry themselves to the point of sleeplessness. The parents will haul the child to one specialist after another, subject him to test after test, drug the poor child senseless and then watch him like a hawk. The child would have a palpable diagnosis, expressible in numerical terms for the purpose of insurance reimbursement. I had nothing of the kind. It is well possible that I simply did not have anything to say at the time. I made up for it later.

I can reach back and dig into those early days of silence. I feel them as times of happy independence, of protection from the inevitable hurt of the raging river of words. It was not as if I was about to get a word in. The ability to speak caught up to me at a certain point, but making myself heard was another matter. I have had opinions for as long as I can remember, but the thread of conversation was beyond my control. My father's opinion was worse than controlling, it was the *only* opinion on subjects that ranged from international politics to whether the next Yankee would hit safely with two outs, driving in a run. Imagine my mouth with a zipper on it and a padlock at one end, as you might see in a cartoon, and then drain all the humor out of the cartoon.

My father got all his information from the New York Times, which he would read cover to cover. He had an unfortunate habit of reading aloud from the paper if something interested or stimulated him, regardless of the conversational trajectory of the other people around him. One day when all we siblings were adults, we sat at the kitchen table, having a conversation. Our father started to read the newspaper aloud. We ignored him. He began again. We continued our conversation without reference to the subject of his fascination. He threw the newspaper down and stormed out of the room like a hurt little boy.

As an older child and then as an adolescent, one of the things that saved me from my father's steamroller was the fact that he was usually out of the house, running his medical practice or running after women. For that matter, my mother was often out of the house, teaching or doing her graduate course work, or if she were home, she would be lying inert somewhere, exhausted and overwhelmed by the basic transactions of life. Housekeepers took care of us. These were African-American women from the south. Some could cook exceptionally well, but all could cook better than my mother, who has never understood the interplay of culinary ingredients and what happens when heat is applied to proteins. Beyond improving the quality of our cuisine, some of these women had the patience to listen to us.

There are occasions as an adult—not often but distinct occasions—when I have to make some kind of moral decision. I do not have an inner parental voice to help me, but one of these black women often shows up just in time. "You know you shouldn't do that," or "that person needs your help." If I have compassion—and it has never been my strong suit—I know where it came from. I have a distinctly hard edge, softened at critical times by this inner voice. I'm ready to have it ripen into something better.

Somewhat parallel to my delayed ability to speak, I did not learn to read in first, second, and the first half of third grade. I do not remember anyone, either parents or teachers, noticing this, but I do distinctly remember discovering books in the middle of third grade and then reading anything I could get my hands on. I was, and am, bookish. I liked history—still do, but my favorite books were atlases. I would pore over atlases for hours. This is silent stuff. Even when we started to take drugs (I say "we" to stress the fact that every one of my friends, bar none, also took drugs), I would curl up with my atlases. When the books by J.R.R. Tolkien became popular, I would imitate the fantasy maps, using markers and paper to create my own inventive worlds. This interior life worked for me. I communicated tangibly with my maps. Verbal articulation was not necessary. My drug friends saw me as some kind of silent sage, communicating on a different plane. We all did lip service to mysticism during that era, perhaps to camouflage the basic fact that what we were doing with drugs was essentially identical with what the generation a few years older than us had been doing with footballs and Corvette Sting Rays. A few of us did not make it, of course—drugs killed then as they do today. I will talk about mind-altering drugs in a later chapter, but the key here is that I gave them up early, before most of the others, because they bored me. I did not need drugs to get into my head—I was already into my head. Vietnam was going on, political assassinations and urban riots, but for a time I had my own survival mechanism.

Despite my vast reading, or perhaps because of it, I was unable to focus on the academic tasks required by high school. I was harassed out of public school for having hair longer than most, and got myself thrown out of one private school after I was caught stealing a chemistry test. After enduring several psychiatric examinations, I was sent to a special private high school, very small, whose main academic requirement was the payment of substantial tuition. The fifteen of us—the entire senior class—majored in sex, drugs, and rock and roll. None of us succeeded in getting ourselves expelled—it just did not happen in that school, although one of us managed to exit by swallowing chlorine bleach. I remember the headmaster assembling us and telling us that it was true, Carl was dead. A few years later, the same headmaster was the subject of a front-page headline in the New York Daily News: "Scandal School: Headmaster was Convicted Child Molester." The state closed the school down. Do not worry—he never got his paws anywhere near me.

I did not go to college right away, but I never stopped reading. I saw all the films of Federico Fellini, Ingmar Bergman, Akira Kurosawa, Jean-Luc Godard, Michelangelo Antonioni, and Francois Truffaut. I went to Europe, met a woman there, and married her. My birth date got a favorable number in the draft lottery. I returned to New York, entered college at age twenty-two, and did very well. I discovered I could write. My brain began to focus. All this time, however, without consulting me, my father remained my father. For the next twenty-five years, I tried to speak with him. My sisters were at it as well, but none of us got anywhere. Oceans of words continued to emanate unedited from his lips, with himself as the usual subject.

The torrent only began to ebb after he got a diagnosis of esophageal cancer. Surgery, radiation, chemotherapy and stents inexorably compromised his ability to shove air out of his windpipe. You could tell that he wanted to say something—preferably something adroitly clever, but nothing could come out.

Sometime during my father's three-year period of decline, my sisters and I were talking about him. "What is he worried about," I remarked, focusing on the man's narcissism. "The world is going to end when he dies anyway." I got an instant guffaw out of one sister, but the other two took an uncomfortably long time to get my meaning. They finally accepted the irony in my statement, but I never said anything like that again about him. I should have remained silent, not to cave in to his bluster, but because it was so sadly waning. He was the only father we had. We could have given him some respect despite himself. It is too late for that now.

My father choked to death just two weeks before the attacks on September 11th. When I watched those events on television, my first thought was "for the first time, he has no unassailable opinion." I could not help having such a self-centered reaction, and I felt awful and numb once I realized that people were jumping out of buildings so they would not be deep-fried in jet fuel. Later that year, at my family's first Thanksgiving dinner without our father, one of my sisters remarked that it was the first family gathering where we were actually having a normal flow of conversation. My mother burst into tears. My father muzzled her for years, so thoroughly that it became second nature. The First Amendment prohibits Congress from abridging your right to speak, but it says nothing about your father. Where your father is concerned, you might have to fight. All four of the siblings fought bravely for the right at one time or another.

I am no child now—my son is now a grown man with three kids of his own—but you never get over the traumas of your childhood. I might have been a little uncomfortable the first time I spoke in front of a group—I recall my throat felt like a cactus—but my fear of being silenced drove me through every barrier. I came to love public speaking. I became a public speaking trainer, and have a public speaking book on the market. My father attended one of my speeches once, and complimented me. That means everything to me.

Now Parkinson's disease compromises my voice. The obstacle is different but the threat is as severe. My ability to write gives me much joy, but it pales in the face of my need to speak my mind. I have a voice in a metaphorical sense, and I need literally to safeguard it.

What do I do about the fact that my voice is fading? My own tactic is to become more deliberate in my speaking, to speak one-on-one as if I were addressing a group, to inject some purposeful formality into the process. It should not be necessary, but I have to do something to bring my voice across. When I say "thank you" to a waiter or a supermarket checker, I use my forceful military voice. I make eye contact and make sure I reach the other person. I do not know about you, but I thank the bagger in the supermarket also. Across a table, I lean in and make eye contact, convinced that the visual connection focuses my voice.

I have not had the occasion to address a group since the Parkinson's process began for me. When I was feeling major body positioning issues, I feared I could not stand straight—a wobbling orator does not command much presence. I visualized myself leaning on my cane, using it as a clever prop. The image failed to gel. The cane is in the closet now. I can once again stand on my own two feet. I have what every speaker needs, a topic. Everybody knows someone with Parkinson's disease. If my body falters, if my voice flags, I can pick myself up, make fun of myself a little, use my challenges as ammunition. If I have to exaggerate, to scream just to seem to speak at a normal volume, I will do what I have to do. The effort I have put into this book demands that I get out in front of community groups to publicize it, focus my body, focus my voice, reach my audience at all costs, in spite of all terror, as any speaker should. Because the vocal power issues remain after many other Parkinson's issues have been resolved, it becomes critically important for me, particularly considering my history of expressing myself. I swear that Parkinson's will not silence me. Silence is the worst form of damnation, the ultimate hell. I cannot help the fact that one day I will be dead, but until that moment, I will not be silent.

*

I have mentioned my three sisters a great deal in this section. They have each had their own issues with both parents (and from time to time with each other), but when I got sick, they were unstinting, united, and effective. It is time I give some space to them.

The people who love you are the people who hear you.

Sisterhood of Caring

Without my three sisters, I would be...no I would not be.

Each of my three younger sisters has a brother with Parkinson's disease. I do not mean here to state a logical or grammatical bit of obviousness, but rather to stress that each sister is involved in some very particular way with the care and support of my body, my mind, and my soul. I doubt a day goes by for any of my sisters in which they do not think of ways to help me, both large and small. My sisters are my core network. I could not imagine living without them.

Being the oldest, I started as an only child, then had a sister, another, a long stretch, and then—was it a half century ago we got the girl we used to call "the baby?" I have the knack of making my sisters laugh uncontrollably, with different triggers and catch phrases for each. In all respects, my relationship with each varies dramatically from my relationship with the others: three distinct tracks. I cherish each.

As the oldest and the only male, I realize I had always lived with the assumption that I would predecease all three of my sisters, they would mourn me when I died, and then follow me in death at the appropriate time. Before Parkinson's but well into middle age, I had a grim epiphany: I could lose one or more of my sisters through disease, terrorism, accident, and the thought was not good. Once this perceptual door was open, I could not close it. The thought of losing any of my sisters is heartbreaking for me. The years abrade them as they decrease me. Death could tease me by stringing me along, and take one of them away while

I am still around. This is the way death has of taking pieces out of you. There is no arguing with it.

My sisters have been hovering around their beloved big brother since the beginning health alarm, as if they knew from a collective sixth sense something was going to happen. They did not know about my early symptoms—I myself did not know what they signified. They first became involved when I was living two thousand miles from them, in Albuquerque, New Mexico, six months into the cycle. One morning, my left leg was weak and in pain, my left arm weak and numb. I had no primary care physician and felt I needed doctors to look at me—that day. My worst fear was a stroke. I knew I had something beyond fatigue. I called 911 and got myself to the University of New Mexico Hospital emergency room. During my fourteen-hour stay, five nurses and doctors tested me separately for stroke, I got an EKG, blood tests, even an echogram to rule out a blood clot, all negative. They diagnosed me with musculoskeletal pain. No one thought of recommending I see a neurologist, and the notion did not cross my mind.

Most of the ER stay consisted of contact with worried sisters, all far away in New York, frustrated at their ability to give me only words, by cell phone and text. Each call from each girl had a distinct coloration, like the timbre of individual musical instruments, and yet the trio performed as if they had smoothly rehearsed. They had indeed been on the phone with each other, and I would not have put it past the youngest sister, Nina, a Broadway producer, to arrange a conference call. Although I was not surprised by the solidarity and support, I was taken by the level of caring. This kind of thing happens when you are so used to being self-sufficient and the moment gives you permission to shove that self-reliance to one side. A dozen years previously, I had had surgery to remove a melanoma from my arm, but I had a wife then. I had never before involved my sisters in my health issues.

Back in my Albuquerque apartment over the next weeks the contact continued. They all bemoaned the many miles between us, I bemoaned it, my health did not improve, I had significant breathing issues, and I decided to leave my beloved mountain to be closer to the ones I loved. Albuquerque, if you cannot go into nature, becomes something like a vast series of tire stores, punctuated by some artistically maintained lane dividers. They even bedeck the freeway interchange with slabs of turquoise and adobe, but without the mountain…just looking at it!

I made the move back to Westchester County, New York where I grew up. Eventually, after seeing an orthopedist, having useless pain treatments and useless physical therapy, I sat in front of my first neurologist (out of three), ready for anything. I brought the MRI from the orthopedist showing I had a bulging disk in my lower spine. The doctor examined me.

"Half the people your age have bulging disks," she said, in her sing-song Indian accent. "The problem is probably in your brain."

"Oh, it is *just* my brain!" I thought, nodding for her to continue.

"It could be a brain tumor," she continued. "It is possible the melanoma from your arm spread up to your brain."

"I had the melanoma removed twelve years ago. The biopsy was clear."

"Let us see," she said.

The doctor sent me for a brain MRI, for starters. I am no Woody Allen worrier, but let us just say the possibility of a brain tumor caused me to clean up some of my affairs and close a few disused online accounts. I also made a strategic list of what I would have to do if…if. If I did get a "serious" diagnosis—and I remembered my father's fatal diagnosis—I would have to involve my sisters in various ways, but until then…

"No. You cannot go alone to get the news," my sister Susie lectured me. "If it's something serious, you might not be able to take it in all at once." I did not argue. We soon sat in front of the doctor, two against one.

"You do not have a tumor," the doctor said in her Indian accent. "Look at your brain, the lesions—it's a mess." At least this is what I heard. My brain has always been something of a mess. Susie's eyes started to mist. I realized after a moment the doctor was saying, "It's MS," meaning multiple sclerosis. She asked me to try to walk around the room. I stumbled and careened. Susie explained how she had been concerned about my gait. Her eyes glistened with unalloyed worry. I felt the total support, the total love. I was thankful I took her suggestion to bring her along. She was right—too much to handle at once, this time, on my own.

The doctor sent me for further tests: two spinal MRIs and a lumbar punch fluoroscopy. I was able to drive myself to and from the MRIs. For the lumbar punch, the minimal need was for me not to drive afterward because of the risk of splitting headaches—and I reacted with a week's worth. Still, I am not squeamish about medical procedures, did not need hand holding, and yet my sisters Nora and Nina insisted on being present through the procedure and the recovery period afterward—about three hours. Nora (a musician and composer) picked me up and drove me in to the hospital, sat with me as I waited in the reception area. Nina came up from work in Manhattan on the train. Here I was, afloat in familial love. I had never realized how very close we all were. Except for the period of the actual procedure, the sisters were with me. Astonishingly, the hospital fed me afterward. The sisters watched with great concern as I picked gingerly at the food, but I got it all down. Tears welled in their eyes. Tears welled in mine. The time finally came when the hospital allowed me to leave. The sun on the top level of the parking structure nearly blinded me, my head began to throb, I held out a sightless hand for an arm to steady myself, an arm appeared, and then another.

A few days later, for the definitive diagnosis, Nora accompanied me to the doctor to help me soak it all in. I remembered sixty years earlier when Nora suddenly appeared to make our cramped family apartment in the Bronx even more cramped. That turned a me into a we, an only child into a big brother. The neurologist said, yes, I had MS, wrote me out a prescription for Copaxone and instructed me on how to inject the drug, Nora hanging on every word. Nora's presence was valuable, because she noticed, and I did not, a dollop of tentativeness in the doctor's voice. Nora mentioned that tentativeness when we were driving back, but my brain was already in gear to get my drugs, follow a special MS diet I already had the book for, join a support group, and start writing a book. I had lacked any diagnosis for a painful and frightening eighteen-month period, and now I could take some action, do something.

Nora kept the observation in storage. Months later, she brought it out into the open when I announced that a second neurologist had changed my diagnosis to Parkinson's disease. You do not get anything by Nora. In an uncertain time, her perspicacity was extremely valuable in pushing me to get the proper diagnosis and treatment.

I am not getting any younger. If I had cancer or a stroke, if I had diabetes or schizophrenia, my sisters, my core constituency, would stay with their big brother. Since my brain is, at least in some manner, "a mess," I always worry that I will suffer cognitive issues, either in addition to the Parkinson's or because of it. If dementia caused me to have worrying symptoms—for example, if I woke up one day a Boston Red Sox fan (especially if I started to talk like one)—my sisters would have an ongoing tragedy on their hands (consoling my son, for one thing), but I know they are tough enough to handle it.

Since getting on the right track with my diagnosis and treatment, I have participated in the Parkinson's Progression Markers Initiative (PPMI) sponsored by the Michael J. Fox Foundation for Parkinson's Research. My sister Susie, who is a comic actress, has volunteered her time to perform at a number of benefits for the Foundation. Susie is an extremely busy person—she always seems to be flying to "the coast"—and she did not get around to telling me she was involved until after the fact, or else she figured I would learn of her involvement by some form of osmosis. I appreciate it in any case. Certainly, we both care about people who suffer from other diseases, but when a health issue touches you, you generally try to do what you can to touch it. When people you love care about you, you have a core, a mooring, a great continuity. You live in the certainty that every moment, even a moment of challenge, is precious.

*

The girls were around when I struggled to begin. They have seen their brother go through many trials, not the least of which, the schoolyard…

As a kid, when you fail in front of others the criticism you imagine is eternal.

Uncoordinated

I grew up in a fog, clumsy and maladroit. Is the Parkinson's disease just a magnification of this?

I have read on numerous occasions that schoolgirls are cruel. They form cliques, jockey for position, and engage in merciless bullying of those girls who do not fit their narrow social templates. I grew into the world as a boy. I did not understand girls. They were nice to look at, but all that girl-ness scattered past me when I was young in a great cackling blur. The girl-world seemed a fortress—you could just make out the outer walls, thickly built and defiant, but the inner realm volunteered nothing. When you grow up to be a man, you come to know a little bit about women, at least enough to coexist with them, but you are still left with the mystery of girls, that private realm women keep under emotional lock and key.

If girls are cruel, I know nothing of it. I only know the abiding meanness of boys. My parents would never admit to pushing me out of the house and into a maelstrom of brutal sadists, otherwise known as an elementary school. They saw it diff… well I cannot imagine how they saw it. The taste of blood still wells in my nostrils. The blood colors pavement and coagulates into flecks that will eventually meld with dirt and return to the earth. There is a sensation when you are attempting to make your way down a path or a street that reeks of menace in the form of hulking human figures on whom you dare not focus. Your blood pulses—this time you are ready to go down swinging, to die trying, but you should not have to risk death, even a small chunk of emotional death, just to get safely into a school. They can tell you are thinking this way, and you can tell, that your non-muscles will not cooperate with your will. You will not coordinate body segments into any meaningful sequence of force. They will get you, and if this were suddenly converted into a real jungle, they would kill you—for the fun of it.

Over the decades, I have undoubtedly magnified and distorted those few times others beat me up, and compressed into a handful those hundreds of schooldays when no incident occurred, but I do not exaggerate when I state that every gym class functioned as a squirm-fest, each attempt at a game or a sport a blazing ordeal. Bar none. In these cases, the other boys do not knock you down (unless it is part of the sport), they judge you, which might very well be more damaging. When your physical blood begins to flow, it coagulates so that you may continue to sustain life. You can take yourself to the school nurse and get some attention, even nurture. By contrast, psychic blood can flow in unlimited quantities. You go into a state of shock from blood loss, and you remain there. No one helps you, because…

…because if you are uncoordinated, you are never right, not to the boys who stare you down with the ardent wish you did not exist, nor to the girls for whom you actually do not exist.

If you are uncoordinated, you are never right. You are never the one betrayed. You are the betrayer, the kid who refuses to play along with the obvious. They do not understand why you cannot accomplish something as simple as connecting a bat to a ball, or, if you manage it, why you run so slowly that the outfielder throws you out at first base after you hit the ball safely, or if you do somehow get to first, why you are still holding onto the bat.

Baseball is the cruelest game boys play. Think of this— when you stand at the plate with a bat, the eight other players on your team have their sixteen eyes focused on you alone. Those waiting behind you want you to hit safely so they can have their turns. Those already on base focus on churning up further real estate, for personal glory and team victory. Your ineptitude threatens both, directly, with no mitigation. To add to this, the other team has nine players who are dedicated to erasing you from the face of the earth. A stream of patter comes out of the catcher, designed to denigrate you and force you to fail in advance. You do not know how to ignore it. You do not like the fact that you were chosen dead last, but if you were doing the choosing you would not argue with the status. You swing and miss. A wave of scorn hits you. You can tell the tone of the jibes but you cannot make out the words for the thumping of blood in the middle of your swirling head. The words blur out entirely and you feel dust on the roof of your mouth. You hear the thump of the ball hitting the catcher's mitt before the pitcher even seems to throw. That makes two strikes. You have got to swing for the next one. In an astonishing moment, you feel the bat making contact with the ball. This time you will not fail them, or yourself. After what seems an eternity, you make the decision that you ought to run for first base. You cannot look at anything except that base, but you sense the easy toss from the pitcher, who has evidently fielded your lame effort, and the equal ease of the first baseman, who has the ball in his glove while you are still half way. No matter, you are going to touch that base even though you are out, but he sees your fool determination and will not allow the gesture. A fuming mess of verbiage assails you. Another groove etches your edifice atilt.

The baseball example is iconic, but it is awash in thousands of other clumsy movements and maladroit sequences that fill the span between your first steps and…well why don't we say…your first kiss (*that* went well, but that's another book, or perhaps a trilogy). I need not go into them individually to make my point. Suffice it to say that if because of Parkinson's disease I have difficulty today opening a door or getting my arms into a jacket, I see this as a worsening of my lifelong lack of coordination instead of something bright shiny and new.

When I first participated in the Parkinson's Progression Markers Initiative (PPMI), sponsored by the Michael J. Fox Foundation for Parkinson's Research, a neurologist examined me extensively on successive days, giving me much more time than my regular neurologist (Neurologist Three). In examining my background, he told me that there has never been any clear correlation between growing up uncoordinated and coming down with Parkinson's later in life. That said, he wanted to do some research into it. The research would be necessarily inexact, since you would have to measure the past lack of coordination of patients you could only examine in the Parkinson's present. You would be depending largely on anecdotal evidence. These people do not have cabinets full of reverse trophies for athletic incompetence. You only have their word for it.

But you can take my word on it. For my entire life, I have walked without any apparent rhythm and have not been able to stand straight without lurching and reeling. Give me a knife, a fork, and a plate of food and I will arrive at only the roughest of results, usually measured by an extra layer of grease on my shirt. There is a positive side to this. I came to Parkinson's (or rather it came to me), with a phalanx of coping mechanisms already in place.

I cannot dance. "That's crazy," someone will tell me, "You only have to have the right instructor." Been there—did that. My wife Monica forced me into many months of dancing lessons, the two of us together. It might have been a coping mechanism, but I could swear I had asthma at the time. Forty-five minutes would leave me completely spent. I am a music lover, and that might have helped me get through it, but every moment of dancing or attempting to look like I was dancing was torture. If someone were to devise a hell for my eternal punishment, it would be a dance at which I was forced against my nature to make myself look like I was enjoying myself. I do not get it, but I know that is because I cannot do it. Yes, it has come to my attention that dance is used as a therapy for Parkinson's. This would be a huge step for me, and I do not mean *that* kind of step. Don't expect me.

As some people dance with automaticity, I cook without thinking of it. I have prepared food all my life (even if I cannot consume it neatly). To the skills and sensitivities I already had, I added a full-time professional degree in baking and pastry some time ago. My attendance at cooking school in fact was the spark that switched me from a business and legal writer to a food and then a wine writer. Parkinson's has not dented my sensitivity to ingredients and my ability to judge and react to the way heat and other environmental forces affects those ingredients. I only have to start slicing an onion to feel a sublime focus, the kind that flees from my grasp so often in my daily Parkinson's life. My theory is that the process of food preparation, which usually starts with aromatic vegetables, activates my deep impulse to be free and independent. I have already written of the way my father pushed me into a realm of silence, but I also had an existential problem with my mother. My mother was a criminal and food was her victim. She could and would denude any edible substance of both flavor and texture. As an aesthetically sensitive boy, I needed to cook for myself to have any sensation of gustatory survival. When the survival mechanism activates, you can wield sharp knives and labor over hot burners without risk of physical harm. If you want to label that "coordination," so be it.

People who can dance, who can shuffle and deal cards with elegance and lightness, who can hit baseballs and tennis balls and golf balls and transfer them to the approximate area where they belong, are by temperament incapable of understanding people who cannot. I do not own dancing shoes, or a tennis outfit, or golf-wear, or anything like that because, as we shall see, just dealing with my regular clothing is struggle enough.

Nudity would certainly be a great thing if you did not have to look at everyone else.

Putting It On, Taking It Off

With Parkinson's, I much prefer near nudity to clothedness, but now and then you have to leave the house.

I love to be naked. Clothing has always pressed upon me. I am difficult to fit. I have short arms and short legs that conspire with a long torso to make shirts pull out, pants slither down. I am hard and lean on most of my body—my arms, legs, chest, back and butt (if you could call that slight protrusion an actual butt)—and yet I carry a layer of fat around my middle that resists thinning with a vengeance. When I find clothing items I like, I wear them to death anything but shop—and then hold onto them until they are useless even as rags. As I write this on a warm and humid evening, I am wearing a pair of boxer shorts—too old to put an origin date on—and a plain white T-shirt, well ventilated by the random erosion of sweat, washing, and wear. Ha—you thought I lounged around in a smoking jacket and ascot. Clothing was difficult for me before, but now with Parkinson's in the mix it becomes a true challenge.

To begin at the beginning, take, for example, underpants. The stock question for a man is, "boxer shorts or briefs." I can answer, "both," although not at the same time. When I am dressed in street clothes, I wear white briefs, for good support. I prefer a French brand called Eminance. They are very expensive but sturdy. When I am lounging about the apartment, I take comfort in my collection of patterned boxer shorts from the Gap. So I cover (or am covered by) what usually can be considered "the two." Of course, as in many areas of this ambiguous life, there are more choices than two: boxer shorts, briefs, long johns, thermals, jock straps, and of course the ultimate choice, no undies at all. I sleep in the boxers. By the way, since I do not consider the boxers underwear, and since they are nicely designed, I will answer the door in them.

The boxer shorts and briefs each present problems relating to gravity, friction, or both. The briefs do not want to be put on and they do not want to be taken off. My first task in putting them on is to get one leg through. I put the left foot in first, easy enough, but for the right foot, I must balance on my shaky left leg. My right foot invariably experiences friction against the seat of the briefs as it seeks the opening. I depend here on my right toes (my right side is the good side) to fine-tune the movement. I might fall if I do not accomplish the maneuver in one quick movement—try, meet resistance, vector the toes, get the right leg through and onto the floor, balance my whole body. To fall when putting on underwear is particularly demoralizing. Of course, I am hardly finished—I now have to pull the briefs up, and they do not want to move up. I grab both right and left sides of the waistband, trying to pull the sides up in one jerk motion, but the stronger right side places itself more successfully than the tentative left side. I never have true confidence in my left hand and arm, but I grab the left side, not fully feeling the grab, and tug up as my right side adjusts. A few more movements on each side and I have the briefs elevated waist-wise, but the crotch remains un-supporting. The right hand pushes the left of the crotch to snugness, but the left hand can only do so much. I declare the process complete, even though I feel I could do much more. Putting a pair of pants on over the briefs might bring a more secure feeling, but often the entire assembly droops.

Boxer shorts—which in my case are intentionally loose wisps—present their own problems. Once I have them oriented fly in front, I need to balance on my right leg to get the left leg into the leg hole without jamming my left foot on the crotch, causing me to either rip the boxers, topple over, or both (it has happened, and those things are expensive). This requires aiming all the toes of my challenged left foot into a scrunched arrow, which I do, but with cerebral rather than tactile confidence. I am never sure of what I am doing or feeling when my left side is involved. I switch legs and quickly get the right foot into the boxers. It is probably a smoother set of movements than it feels to me, but I am never confident. It remains to pull up the sides of the boxers to my waist, which seems simple enough, except that I need to see my upward progress because I cannot truly feel it. My first effort brings them up to my hips, I feel a wave of exhaustion, I try a second pull-up and worry that my left side is not keeping up with the right, and I usually need a third effort to get the boxers well situated around my waist.

Now it is time for a shirt. These come in several varieties, T, polo, and button-down. In putting on a T-shirt, it is the gossamer lightness of the thing—its most desirable attribute when the shirt is actually on my body—that provides the challenge. First, I need to fight with the folds of the shirt—they have a mind of their own—to ascertain by some scrap remnant of a label which end is back and which is front. Once I do this, I need to correctly orient the shirt so I can attempt to get my head into it and, I hope, find an exit for each arm. Once I succeed in filling the three holes in proper orientation, the T-shirt will invariably cling across my chest. I must muster every bit of potential concentration to fight against the friction that keeps it where I do not want it, rolling my challenged fingers against the insides of the shirt bottoms until gravity finally relieves the tension. A good shake of my body cements the relationship. A polo shirt is somewhat easier because of the collar, which aids in orientation, and the somewhat thicker fabric, which nicely invokes the law of gravity. A button-down shirt, long sleeve or short, is less of a problem. The buttons are not easy but I take them one at a time.

Long trousers pose the same challenge they did before I had Parkinson's: getting into them without tripping. Here I do sit down, get my legs through, and only stand when I feel a solid, definite, unencumbered bond between my feet and the floor. Getting a shirt tucked in and fastening the waist before the shirt tucks itself out takes a level of muscular coordination I never knew I had until I lost it. I need to leave my pants unfastened to give myself room to tuck in the shirttails. Gravity will then claim the loosened pants and I will have to try to catch the sides with the heels of my hands, quickly fasten the front of the pants, and then exert a supreme effort to adjust the shirttails within the waistband. The zipper remains. I need to use my left hand to buttress the flaps of the fly so I can assure a smooth, snag-free path for the closing movement. Getting all these things done requires a degree of simultaneity I find I now lack. Multi-tasking is not the Parkinson's way.

Putting on a pair of shoes incites both my balance problem and the weakness I endure in my left arm and leg. The left foot gives the real problem. I prefer shoes with laces for the support they give. I use a sturdy metal shoehorn for support and guidance. Because I lack feeling in my left foot and lower leg, I have trouble coordinating left foot, shoehorn and shoe together and often can only nestle the shoehorn around the outside of the left heel, leading to an insecure positioning and necessitating a great deal of wriggling. My right shoe is straightforward. From a sitting position, I can bend down to tie my right shoe, but cannot do this with my left without pain and the onset of trembling in my torso. I need to cross my left leg over my right knee to get the shoe tied, and this movement activates pain, tingling, and weakness in my entire left side. My solution to this is entirely a sense of purpose. I do it—I simply do it, but I am not happy about it.

Once the colder weather comes, I need to get into and out of a coat. I approach this task weak left arm first. I need to get my left arm all the way into the sleeve at first try because the arm lacks the coordinated power to push its way through with the force necessary to get my hand and wrist through the elastic cuff. Once I get through the coat friction to slide the arm in, I pull on the left cuff with my right hand to adjust. I then need to contort my body so the right edges of the coat do not bunch up around my back. Given that the coat is now pivoting from my left side, I might need several attempts to find the right armhole. When I do, I thread my right hand and arm into the right sleeve, although here I do have pushing power. I take a moment to center myself before I move on to the task of zipping up the coat. In removing the coat, I get my right hand out first and then use the right hand to hold onto the left cuff and coordinate the extraction of my left arm. I finally muster the balance I need to hang the coat on a chair. I find the coat process so trying that if I visit someone for a short while, I often steam in the coat rather than remove it only to have to get into it again.

I enjoy dressing up in jacket and tie, but I rarely get the chance. Just three days after I switched from the MS medication to the Parkinson's medication, I got my chance—my niece's Bat Mitzvah. Try as I might, I could not knot the tie, but after much thought, I concluded that I had simply forgotten how to do the knot. Later, after attending the event with open collar (I was not the only one) I placed myself in front of a mirror and after half a dozen attempts got the job done. I must have tied a tie ten thousand times over the course of my life, forgotten, and remembered. I forced myself to ascribe the difficulty to anxiety and insisted that Parkinson's disease had nothing to do with it. You might be evil, but you do not touch me everywhere!

*

Wait a second. My phone is ringing. It is somewhere snug inside that jacket. Now how do I get to it and handle all that finger contact before the caller gets sent over to voice mail?

Despite the Emancipation Proclamation, we are all slaves...to our smart-phones.

My Big Fat Smart Phone

Operating a smart phone is a surprisingly athletic activity.

When I traded in my compact, fits-in-the-palm-of-your-hand dumb-phone for my so-big-you-can-defend-yourself-with-it smart-phone, I already had Parkinson's disease, I just didn't know it (and would not know it for another two years). Initially I went smart phone for a better camera after missing a photo of a bear in the Sandia mountains, but as you can guess (because it has probably happened to you), I became instantly transfixed by the smart-phone capabilities, especially the ability to surf the web through Wi-Fi. Without the device, how could I force other people to look at photos of my adorable grandchildren at every stage in their development?

I am profoundly right-handed. This actually means I hold the phone in my left hand, so I can use the phone's stylus with my right. Character entry by hand on a phone is beyond me. I use the stylus to enter letters, numbers, and symbols one precise character at a time. Fortunately, the phone is first rate at guessing the next word I am trying to enter—"birthday" after "happy," for example. I was impressed when it prompted me for the full nickname I use when writing to one of my sisters after I entered just the first two letters. My phone is smart, and seems to be getting smarter. My level of intelligence at best remains the same. Which one of us do you think will win this race?

Early in the relationship, when using the phone to play my beloved Spider Solitaire, I would recline on my couch, holding arms, left hand and heavy phone suspended strategically above my face. When I began to feel pain, weakness and tingling in my left arm and hand, I first blamed the weight of the phone for the symptoms. The difficulty seemed a small price to pay for such electronic joy. If you are not addicted to a cellular phone game, you might not understand. It is not a drug—there is no such thing as an official overdose. The time came when I realized I could have some kind of musculoskeletal or neurological disorder. It took weeks before "could have" morphed into "probably have," and even longer for me to look into what the problem could be. Parkinson's was creeping in on me, stealthily. The bottom line was that holding the phone in my left hand was getting to be more and more of a muscle and coordination problem.

In writing or answering e-mails on the phone, I tap one character at a time with the stylus. Rather than frustrate me, this repeated action serves to assert my connection with that extension of my personality others call a mere phone. There is nothing "mere" about my phone. Steal it from me and I will contemplate the emergency room, where I will demand a sedative. If I forget the phone…there is no if—it never happens. I never forget the thing and I am always aware of its location, even its top-bottom orientation. There are certain parts of my body that I treasure more than I do the phone, but not many.

I use the phone to check in at restaurants using social media. The restaurants do not like all this activity, posting and picture snapping, since it hogs up tables longer, but no, that is not my responsibility. If I want to check in and let my family and friends know about my chicken fajitas that is my own indulgence. The process brings me closer to the phone in an environment in which I probably will have to put the phone aside for other utensils. During the main segment of the meal, I will have to put the phone away, satisfying myself with an occasional tap on its protrusive outline in my clothing as if I were secretly giving myself sexual arousal (which in some sense, probably, I am). The all-important stylus rests sheathed, but its quivering potency is never far from my consciousness, except when I am drinking wine, which takes precedence over the phone (and much else). I ought to add that having a beautiful woman as my dining companion will serve the same purpose, although here the wine, let us freely admit, also tends to help. I have an abiding interest in wine, women and song. Where do I keep a handy repository of songs? You guessed it: on my phone. How do I keep in touch with women, e-mail them, photograph them? Phone, of course. How do I track down vintages? Yup. So my interests and leanings boil down from wine, women and song to phone, phone and phone.

Using the phone to make and receive calls creates its own special set of coordination challenges. I need my right hand to operate the thing and yet my left hand trembles, despite the medication—it trembles even now as I type. Since the left hand is subject to some degree of motion, the right hand and fingers need to coordinate like aircraft landing on a carrier deck. When receiving a call I need to swipe rightward across a green circle to answer, and this invariably takes more than one attempt. I need then to poke my right index finger to activate the speakerphone feature, which is the only way I can actually hear the other person. This is not because of any hearing loss on my part but because of equipment volume limits that conform to hyper-strict European Union regulations designed to protect people's hearing. Once connected, I may then switch the phone to my stronger right hand. The left hand, the Parkinson's hand, floats when I leave it free, so I have to find some place to put it or something to do with it. It is not as if I can scratch my nose with the left fingers, since I truly do not feel the tactile contact. Left hand scratching through fabric is even less successful. If I can sit on the left hand or get it into a pocket, that works.

Dialing a new number presents a range of dexterity challenges. I need my reading glasses to read a number from a computer screen or scrawled on a piece of paper. I need my reading glasses to focus on the numbers I am pressing. The phone is still in my left hand as I tap speakerphone. I use my right hand to remove the glasses and get them somewhere secure, hoping to switch the phone to my right hand before I get an answer. If I think of it and the call is to a business that might have a phone menu, I also quickly hit the screen button so the number pad once again shows. All these quick moves in rapid sequence leave me but a split second for the thinking part of my brain to catch up to the operations portion. Suffice it to say I try to get through the call as quickly and efficiently as possible so I can lie down or have a drink. Calls to my contact list, especially to regular people, are a little more straightforward, taking fewer steps.

With Parkinson's I tend to do things in discrete stages, where, before Parkinson's, I might have combined them into more fluid sequences. I am never free from the concern that the phone will sap or exhaust a limited resource, be it dexterity, energy, the ability of my eyes to focus on the screen, or that all-important consideration, remaining battery life. I am certain that if William Shakespeare were alive and writing today, he would factor remaining battery life into his plays—there is potential dramatic material here for both comedies and tragedies. "Methinks that four percent alone to mortal life remains/the glow wanes such that voice mail at the tone scant message holds." As batteries improve, the basic drama of the thing will of course decay. The natural extension of this will be the day when we plug ourselves into the phones and they will transfer energy to us. The ultimate invention would be of course the dopamine phone. I will gladly trade up to that one.

Look, pain—I have work to do. Go bother the neighbors.

Creaky

Broken and leaky, fragile not agile

I am going to keep this section short and bitter.

Years ago, I wrote a musical comedy that, among other lyrical gems, includes a plaintive song in waltz tempo entitled "Creaky."

> Creaky, creaky, broken and leaky
> That's what you get, you can never forget you are
> Older, older, easily colder
> Counting each day, as it all slips away, till the
> Time to check out comes so close
> Sa - yo - na – ra, A - di - os
>
> Fragile, fragile, no longer agile
> Every joint aches with the trouble it takes just for
> Walking, walking, thinking and talking
> Every consumer succumbs to the rumor that
> Life will bring what it will bring
> Life is no forever thing

The theme is, of course, aging, but it might as well be Parkinson's disease. In my case, the two challenges seeped into my consciousness at about the same time. I use the term "consciousness" deliberately. In the case of old age (the question of senior citizen discounts aside), it takes time to admit to yourself and others that you have gotten there. In the case of Parkinson's disease, it is often the case, and it was my case, that the disease precedes the diagnosis by years, maybe even by a decade or more. As Dr. James Parkinson writes:

"So slight and imperceptible are the first inroads of this malady, and so extremely slow is its progress, that it rarely happens that the patient can form any recollection of the precise period of its commencement."

Because of this aspect, it is not always easy to tell the difference between Parkinson's creakiness and the plain vanilla creakiness I might have regardless.

I cannot claim that my whole body aches all at once, but I do have days where all the individual musculoskeletal systems in their turn bring me pain, stiffness, and distress. Parts of my body snap and clunk when I move, others throb with the Parkinson's shakes, yet others buckle and bend. I merely report this—this is not a complaint. I would not be writing any of this if I felt I did not have the skill to put it in a positive light. If I allowed pain to have final sway, I would do better to condense this book into three powerful words: "I give up." I certainly do not give up. That creaky feeling is nothing else but the overhead of life. As in business, you factor in overhead as you engineer your profit. The machine creaks, you oil it, you get on with the creative process.

You may be thinking, why doesn't he take "something" for the aches and pains? I do take some ibuprofen on occasion, but have not made it a habit. As it is, I take Parkinson's medications three times a day. Three dosages a day seems about the visceral limit to me. I have never had clear evidence that analgesics work for me except when I get a headache, and headaches are fortunately not my problem. I might have my own set of addictions in a metaphorical sense, but substances have never taken hold of me. Opiates may in fact send the pain to some other dimension, but unlike the addict, I dislike the way they make me feel.

A modest dose of alcohol sometimes does work to deaden pain, or at least to make pain easier to bear, especially when my entire body seems to hurt. The problem with alcohol as a painkiller is that it takes the edge off perception just as it takes the edge off the pain. Unlike many of the writers in the American model—I think of Hemingway, Faulkner, and my favorite, Scott Fitzgerald—in exchange for not having alcohol as an illness, I cannot access alcohol as a muse. As a non-alcoholic, alcohol is good for me, but it does nothing for my writing. I do write about wine and spirits professionally, but this is dry work indeed—I fill the glass only after I fill the page. The dry brain is the one that lubricates pages with words. Words fermenting in my heart and mind are more powerful to me than grapes fermenting in a vat. This is true even if those words express pain.

The most consistent pain I endure is the burning and throbbing that engulfs my left calf and shin. One cause is a bulging disk in my lower spine, but my Parkinson's left side disturbance makes the left leg pain worse. This pain is at its worst when I am lying down, a position which otherwise eases most of my other body annoyances. I shift my legs, crossing and re-crossing my ankles, but to no avail. The only way I deal with this pain—my only choice—is to concentrate on it, convert it into an intellectual concept, tell the brain, "Yes, I understand what you are trying to tell me, I have gotten the gist, but you do not have to keep repeating yourself?"

Sometimes—now more often than not—pain listens to me. If I starve it of emotional attention, it slinks off, whimpering, not out the door but at least into a corner. It is lurking there now, but I am going to work on something else now that I have finished this section.

Blues and rock and roll—music with corners—
snug brain coverings—equilibrium

Rock and Roll Just Doesn't

Down with a case of the blues, and no way to turn it into song.

I am a Certified Specialist of Wine, but a man cannot live by wine alone. You need to add women and song to make the time-honored trilogy. I will cover the subject of women later. My vast experience with women has yielded so little insight that perhaps I will boil it all down to a haiku, but even seventeen syllables might be too much to fill. I have escaped hubris by admitting this, so I will move on to song. Music has always been important to me.

I am a good pianist, blues and jazz, but a hot electric guitarist, blues and rock. I know all the chords and jazz theory on the piano, but on the guitar all this eludes me—I just know how to wail, and have been at it since the Kennedy administration. I grab onto the neck of my jet-black Paul Reed Smith solid body guitar and bend strings to make that baby sing. Did I just write, "I grab?" The past tense, "grabbed," is now necessary. With Parkinson's I now lack the athletic strength to wobble the thing with my left hand, to sustain a bent string and finesse into a wondrous array of tone, the fingers do not press, and even chords fade into the distance of memory. Proper medication has given me better movement in many aspects of my life—handling house and car keys, dining out at a restaurant, extracting a credit card from my wallet—but it has not given me my guitar chops back. A truly important segment of my persona is at risk. In the past, I might have neglected my guitar out of inertia, but the knowledge that I *could* wail never ceased to give me a little swagger. Many amateur and even professional guitarists are chords only, but I am a single-string melody man, and of that I am proud. Strap me into a guitar and plug it into an amplifier, and I am alive.

Back to the past tense: I *was* alive. The guitar now seems more a weight than a vehicle for uplifting. I stumble over the thick black case often.

All my blues acumen and pride aside, I turned away from the blues more than ten years ago. I had a long talk with myself and noted several key truths. I have never picked cotton, been in jail, bummed out on skid row. I have university diplomas and journalism awards on my wall. I speak French. I speak grammatical English. I have no right to sing the blues. Feeling a music-lifestyle disconnect, I turned from guitar blues to jazz on the piano with the aim of coming more into line with the sophisticated cocktail pianist I felt was a truer representation of my personality. I studied jazz theory, chords and scales. I wrote eighteen songs for a musical comedy using a lot of that theory. I still picked up the guitar now and then…"picked up," once again that sad past tense, but I had a new sense of my musical self, and I felt comfortable with it. I will always choose the caviar over the grits, the Bordeaux over the Two Buck Chuck.

My sociologically-based "I am no hypocrite" harshness against the blues eased over the years, but left one sticking point—I have already mentioned it—grammatical English. I cannot seem to abandon the chalice of English just to appear hip, even if this rather limits my means of accessing the spirit of the blues.

I write blues songs, and will give you one very soon, using some semblance of good English, but let me first analyze a particular line which has rankled me for years. Guitarist Stevie Ray Vaughan had a hit with the song *The Sky Is Crying* (the African-American original was by Elmore James).

I've got a real, real bad feelin'
That my baby, she don't love me no more

Look at the first line. So *how* bad are you feeling, Stevie
Ray? "Really" bad—that's an adverb—expresses what you
are trying to say, modifying the adjective "bad." The
adjective "real" here is misused (although it is so widely
misused as to lead some commentators to believe it will
one day poke its way into accepted usage as an adverb).

The second line poses three problems. He uses the
improper verb conjugation "don't" where he really means
"doesn't" and adds an unnecessary "no" before "more" (or
"mo" in his parlance), creating a double negative. As if this
were not enough, he employs a double subject. He uses the
noun—"my baby"—and despite this is compelled to
reinforce the subject with the unnecessary pronoun, "she."
At this point, we already know he is singing about his (soon
departing) baby. Oh wait. It just hit me why he stresses the
"she"—gender specificity. Blues is hyper-macho, and he
does not want you to think for a moment that the
aforementioned "baby" could be anything but female, thus
rendering the singer…you know. That must be it.

And so what follows is my grammatical blues song. As for
the baby in question, think what you will. Here is the verse:

Hey pretty baby put your mind at ease
Hey pretty baby put your mind at ease
Can't dance with a guy who has Parkinson's disease

Hey pretty baby let me sit this one out please
Hey pretty baby let me sit this one out please
Can't dance with a guy who has Parkinson's disease

Any effective blues song needs what we call a bridge:

I think I'll swallow Levodopa
Take some Selegiline too
Despite my fondest hope I
Know I can't keep up with you

And then let us polish it off with a closing verse:

I teeter and totter with a weakness in my knees
I teeter and totter with a weakness in my knees
Can't dance with the guy who has Parkinson's disease

Now that I have established the linguistic theme, it is time for a bit of screaming lead guitar, but the fingers of my left hand will not do the bidding of my brain. For me, with my guitar, to paraphrase Mick Jagger, I can't get any satisfaction.

Back to my piano. The Hanon exercises I have known since childhood are designed to build finger dexterity to enhance pianistic ability. They now have quite the opposite effect: I use the touchy-feely relationship I have with my piano with Hanon to strengthen my compromised left hand and fingers to improve my general dexterity away from the keyboard. It is not just strength, but using the hand and fingers with a coordinated elegance I once took for granted. While I may have a feeling of accomplishment, even progress, when I do these routines, I still cannot feel confident when I pick up a glass of water with my left hand. I do not spill the liquid, but cannot escape the feeling that I am about to spill it as the lightened hand strains to float beyond my reach. That hand and the fingers on it will not listen to the commanding brain, because the disease now makes the rules.

Finger exercises are methodical. Real jazz on the piano is melodic and harmonic: labyrinths of minor sevenths relating to dominant sevenths transmuting to major sevenths, and then either exploring the insides of a key or modulating through a relative minor to another key. In the primitive self-taught way I play, the left hand lays down all this structure with the right hand taking care of melody, accent and improvisation. Parkinson's disease compromises my left hand and makes finger movement difficult. The left hand wants to make the right hand wait, while the right hand steams in the agony of a young man's impatience. The two sets of fingers, which used to work as a scrunched together team, are now at odds. The musical brain in the middle knows the song—Cole Porter, Jerome Kern, Rodgers and Hart—but despite all its aesthetic force and passion for song, the brain cannot command the physical left hand to do what it does not want to do. The chain of command is broken. For some reason, the music of Brazilian composer Antônio Carlos Jobim coordinates better for me—"The Girl From Ipanema" with its evanescent bridge, "Desafinado," "Corcovado," "Wave," the brilliant "Waters of March"—I give the composer credit for the ease of melodic and harmonic flow. Perhaps if I started speaking Brazilian Portuguese I could develop a section of my brain that would be free of Parkinsonian inroads.

I have small hands. Before Parkinson's I stressed my hands to the limit to get my music done: splaying, spindling, scrunching fingers into chord voicings, minimizing left hand movement, leaving vast stretches of keyboard undisturbed. My concentration had been the song, that quintessence of language and music I consider the apex of human art. I etched songs into my brain, and, indeed, wrote my own. You are hit with a sad reality when you can no longer interpret the great songs, when left and right sides seem to belong to different pianists, but your reality becomes all the more dismal when you forget the changes in your own songs, even if you do remember the words you wrote. I admit my own songs do not rise to the celestial heights of the greats, but I worked on them hard, they rise automatically in my brain and in my heart, and yet one of my hands will not cooperate with the heart. It is fortunate that I have them all on mp3.

If music and my illness combine to teach me anything, it is the value of listening. I have always listened to music, but I find that lately I have been adding people, and, you know what, they are surprisingly interesting. Where have I been?

To listen is to find another way to speak

A Better Listener

The disease gives me a challenge, and I accept.

PD commonly stands for Parkinson's disease, but it also stands for personal damage. I came to PD with significant PD. It is not enough that I have a book to show for either flavor of PD—it is time to take care of the PD so I can better handle the other PD. I stick my neck out here. I am making a vow. It is time I learned to listen.

Recently on a social media site, I joined a debate on nomenclature raging among some of my food and wine friends. A person who operates a restaurant is a "restaurateur," we all established. The term is derived from the original French *restauration*, meaning "that which restores." The word "restauranteur," with that extra "n," is technically wrong. My spell checker flags it, after all. I gave the matter some thought. My old self would have rallied to the cause of the n-less original. My old self was quick to demonstrate cultural refinement. My old self had a hole in it, however. It was undiplomatic and too direct. People got the hard edge of it. The plain fact is, restauranteur, with that extra "n," is a useful term to denote someone who runs a restaurant. To English speakers, it makes more sense than the original. No one doubts what you mean when you use it. My comment on the social media site was to the point: "I have been pedantic all my life," I wrote, "and what has it gotten me? The extra 'n' is harmless." Several people stood firm on the original, but others agreed with me. The overhead on nit picking what other people are saying is that you hear the delivery, but in exchange you fail to grasp the content. If somebody is talking about a restauranteur, I am better off listening to what they have to say about the restaurant owner than bemoaning the loss of that silly little "n."

Dale Carnegie once wrote, "You can't win an argument."
Agree as I might, I have not followed this precept. Being
right usually means you lose…something. It is time to
change, and to change I need to learn to not only shut my
mouth, but also to put my fiery brain on hold. It is not
going to be easy.

"I can't stand your pedanticism," a friend once told me.
"You mean pedantry," I replied. I see several definitions:
"excessive concern with minor details and rules," "undue
display of learning," "the ostentatious display of academic
knowledge." This is exactly what I did to poor Stevie Ray
Vaughan in the previous section. I am guilty, but I
understand how it all came about. When I was young, I had
to fight for conversational space in the face of my father's
vocal typhoon. He had that need to be right. I could not out-
shout him, but I had a talent for detail (an essential attribute
for a pedant). As an adult, I would use it for a quick thrust
to leave him silent and wounded, be it grammar,
pronunciation of foreign languages, or historical detail. "It
was James Knox *Polk* who was president during the
Mexican War, not Franklin *Pierce*." "You mean baptismal
font, not *fount*." "That skier is from *Slovenia*, not
Slovakia—the two countries don't even border each other."

I cut down my own father. That was not right. He cut me
down. That also was not right. He could not help it. I could
not help it. It would not matter so much, if I had not kept up
the cutting down with other people, who did not have our
biological stake in the matter. I am not the first person to
use illness as a vehicle for personal progress. My father,
however, did not open up during his three-year cascade
from diagnosis to death. You will not find me making the
same mistake. Illness can teach you. Illness can change

you. I have too long been fighting a war. I declare an
armistice, now, before all the land is laid waste.

When you come to think of conversation as a form of
combat, and look at your intellect as armament and armor,
you do not develop a fully rounded set of listening skills.
Growing up, I had known only menace. I had no experience
of healthy conversational interplay, or even the notion that
it had any value. Self-absorbed, with a poor grasp of social
nuance, I existed in a self-contained box. On occasion,
another person would bring my attention to the problem.
More often, the person would just shut me out and shift
their attention elsewhere. People are not impressed that you
are right. They have an understandable desire to protect
themselves from your verbal aggression. You do not see it
as aggression—you just see it as being smart. The body
builder does not hide his musculature, so why should you
dampen your intellect? You do because it is not always
useful. If you stress everything, you effectively stress
nothing. Communication requires editing.

I have a truly sensitive ear when it comes to listening to
music, but over the years, I have been singularly tone deaf
to the voices of other people. I have always known other
people were out there. I mean, there they were, buzzing all
around, the vast majority of them concerned with things
that did not interest or stimulate me: their cars and boats,
their doggies and kitties and that kind of thing. Listening to
them seemed a useless exercise. I had heard of listening
skills. I had even run a Toastmasters Club workshop on
listening skills, but I just did not get it. What I did not get
was the fact that real conversation is not war—it is
connection and a form of love. I perceived their
conversational forays as attacks. My best approach was to
shore up my fortress. I was looking at human interplay as a

zero-sum game—either I did the speaking or they did—there could be no middle ground.

As I slathered decades onto my life, the fortress began to crumble and decay. A point came when I knew that nobody cared how thick my walls were, how well trained my troops. They avoided frontal assault, or any assault—they simply passed me by. I felt an abiding sense of damage. I had the perspective to understand, however, that the bare desire to listen would not be enough. I lacked skills that most people take a lifetime to acquire. What to do?

I will get there. The first step is to undermine the ramparts of my castle and fill in the moat, use fallibility and vulnerability as assets, allow the outside world to rush in and hope that I can find a role to play in the drama. I am no longer the center of the equation. There is no center. There is no equation. We are all in this thing called life together. Everyone depends on everyone else. Having the disease has at least taught me that.

When you fall flat on your face you do not defy the law of gravity, you prove it.

Gravity—It's a Law

You feel small when cosmic forces dispute your getting across a room.

When my keys slip from my hand, they rapidly hit the ground. I have an instant concern that I have (again) damaged the remote entry device for my car—these things are surprisingly expensive to repair. The law of gravity, unlike the laws of the state of New York, is not subject to appeal. Before Parkinson's, I took the limitations and benefits of gravity as a given, never giving the subject much thought. To Parkinson's-me gravity takes on multiple layers of meaning. On the one hand, it is an intensification of a force I have been fighting my entire life, while on the other hand, it is something on which I can no longer rely.

When I stand still, as on a sidewalk waiting for a pedestrian signal, I feel the bad gravity pull me down and the good gravity weaken its grip. This is mostly perception, of course. My sense is that some outside force pulls me rearwards. I reel, shuffle side-to-side, and adjust. I have never fallen outside my home, but I am also never free of the fear that someday it will happen. Passers-by will rush to my aid, calling public attention to what I see to be my private challenge. My body is compact and I am unlikely to suffer more than a few scrapes, but if they ask me if I am all right, I will answer: no, things are not all right, but I cannot easily explain—here, read the book.

In private, walking a few steps across a room involves a lurch or a lunge. I perceive the gravity, swirl around in imbalance, stagger to where I want to go, and then arrest the movement. My body stops but my inner ear and balance center reverberates a moment. Once the event is truly complete, I acknowledge its finish, and move on to the next event. I read a lot about modern physics and its triumph of discontinuity, but I do not want to be the example they use to prove it: "You see how these subatomic particles lurch between states of being, just like a man with Parkinson's disease taking a walk." I do want to continue my walks, not to prove any laws of physics, but to get some air and sun. I use a cane—it helps. Once I get my hooves moving, however, I cannot just do the process, I need to overanalyze it. Most people keep the calculus they use to navigate spaces in the background. Mine is glaring foreground.

Nothing about Parkinson's is automatic. You operate the body using a manual transmission and without power steering. I have referred to gravity as "something on which I can no longer rely." We rely on the law of gravity to keep us from floating up into the stratosphere, and yet I feel poorly connected to the ground, even when I sit. The up, down and sideways pulls on my body do not mathematically or logically reconcile, and yet they coexist. My body reacts to the gravity pulling me in towards the center of the earth by fatiguing all too rapidly, but my brain counters with upward float. I have lived at high altitudes and climbed to even higher altitudes, and it is not pretty gasping for oxygen. Although the altitude rise I feel when I float upwards at sea level is only in my brain, there is no "only" when it comes to my brain. My body feels brain reality as if it is body reality. I know the difference, but I do not live the difference.

Body and brain combine fitfully when I need to carry things. Items swing—coats from my body or bags that I carry—adding a lateral dimension, a pulling and spreading out, until I fear I come close to invading the space of others. I need to cross a major street to bring my wash to the local service laundry. I can hang the bag over my back like Santa's toy sack, but the bag pushes itself and my body from side to side as I walk. I feel this tug first in one foot and then in the other—not good when I need the feet for balanced locomotion. I switch the bag to my left hand, but I never feel a good grip with the left. My right hand takes the brunt of the punishment, but this means I must use my left arm and left side to push open the resistant door of the launderette. Once I do, the pendulous swing of the bag vaults me into the shop after it, and I am lucky I do not lose it completely. I know to anticipate the balance shift, although, even here I can overreact.

Gravity is never absent, for good or ill. With Parkinson's disease, my energy is finite, and gravity tries to scallop out the supply. When I put on a pair of socks and need to gyrate and contort them into place, energy flees. When I attempt to coax a sheaf of broccoli into a produce bag at the market and I need to brace myself against something architectural, energy departs beyond the hope of return. Even typing these words into my computer involves a struggle in which gravity plays a major part. As I sit now, I am bobbing up and down, making constant adjustments as I hunt for the keys I need to generate words. The brain wants to formalize its words, but it must translate the desire through the manifold of a gravity-laden body. My good right leg tends to float up with my body, while my bad left leg plods and sticks into the ground. I am now weary of gravity. We make a poor marriage, but there is no way I can get this one annulled.

The phrase "anxiety attack" does not do justice to the enemy. It is more a total war.

Anxiety

Comes with the Parkinson's territory

The medical profession tells me virtually nothing about anxiety and depression in Parkinson's patients. They are never very clear as to whether you feel anxiety or depression because of some chemical brain imbalance, because of the understandable fact that you worry about having a serious brain disease, or as a side effect of medication. They have a notion that the neurotransmitter serotonin regulates sleep, appetite and mood just as the neurotransmitter dopamine in the brain regulates muscle movement, but they soon run out of science.

This is my brain this time, and I will make the definitions and draw the distinctions. Let us begin with my take on depression. Depression is an interrupt in the ability to process and give value to time as represented by the three units of yesterday, today, and tomorrow. Yesterday was unfortunate. It gave you an opportunity, now forever gone, to create something, to add a bit of light to your life. You allowed it to pass you by, you lost it, but to make matters worse, other people—in this town, on the other side of the county, in China—experienced happiness and joy yesterday, babies were born smiling into the world, billions lived, worked, interacted, loved, and slept without concern. Today, you awoke to discover this dichotomy between a world that radiates hope and light and your own existence, which can only read about these things. Today, you are frozen, impotent to clear out any of the gloom, because there is simply too much of it. Theoretically, you can start with a clean slate tomorrow, but you have no reason to think tomorrow will be any different (if it ever comes). Your concept revolves around the worst. The fact that billions of people live in constant fear of war, political repression, hunger and disease, and you do not, does nothing to allay your despair. Among these billions live the happy ones, the cheerful souls you envy and despise. You saw a trite saying once on a plaque in a gift shop: "There is no way to happiness. Happiness is the way." You buy neither the concept nor the plaque.

There is an abiding certainty in depression, even if the "facts" about which you are certain have no bearing on reality. You have heard of hope, you may even do it lip service, but in truth you are convinced that it cannot find you, much less rescue you. Depression is an infection of belief. It travels in only one direction—down.

Anxiety is something else entirely. In anxiety, the brain has no docking station, nothing firm to hold. Everything, as the early Greek philosopher Heraclitus tells us, is in a constant state of flux. Anxiety at its worst makes you feel overwhelmed, afraid, worried, but at the back of it all there is the notion that you could theoretically do something about it, if only you could find out what it is. You tend to pay excessive attention to details, believing that you can solve the problem by breaking it down into its constituent parts, but like the Hydra of Greek myth, every time you cut off one of the monster's heads, two grow back. Anxiety cycles around itself and feeds on itself. Anxiety causes the shakes, Parkinson's causes the shakes, and it is difficult to know how much of one and how much of the other is causing the shakes.

To confuse matters even more, depression often causes episodes of concomitant anxiety and anxiety brings on concomitant depression. One or the other is usually the main squeeze. In my case, it is anxiety. Doctors diagnosed me with anxiety and treated me for it on two occasions: twenty years ago and ten years ago. The first period was definitely before I had any touch of Parkinson's disease, the second period probably before. I know anxiety when it appears; I also know that when I get that down feeling, it is at worst concomitant depression—whatever you call it, it is not the "Black Dog" Churchill suffered. It is typically a matter of an hour or two. A sandwich, a glass of wine, or a trip to the gym usually takes care of it.

Anxiety and I play a different duet. It might be that the restless feeling that makes me pace the room, organizing my thoughts, is a form of anxiety. This is up to interpretation—you could call it my expression of energy. I am a pacer. I move around when I think. At the computer, I force myself to rise frequently. I might do this in the middle of a sentence, intend to pace around the room, only to find myself bending over the keyboard balancing on the balls of my feet, stooped down and entering text, too unwilling to re-commit my unpadded bottom to my desk chair. I do not call that kind of thing anxiety, because I have had the real thing, the spigot that spews terror for weeks, with no palliative other than chemically-encouraged sleep. This species of anxiety takes its time to appear, building as sand accretes onto a beach, bit by steady bit, until the moment comes when you thought you were safely on shore, but you have been in fact funneled out to sea. Anxiety has an undertow. If you struggle against it, you only exhaust yourself.

Twenty years ago, I was worried about—what do you worry about?—money. I was living in Westport, Connecticut at the time, a town associated with   what is the word?—oh yes, money. I was not one of those people who contributed to the average income or net worth of that community. I had just separated from my wife, Monica. I lived in a basement apartment. One evening I went to a singles event. I met a woman I will call Sharon. She was needy, in the process of separating from her husband, still living with him, with two children in the middle. I have a weak spot for vulnerability. It makes me feel like a leader, strong, like Caesar. Here—let me protect you with my cloak. Leave everything to me. The woman did so. Our desire was extreme, the chemistry explosive. I went with the flow on that one, welcoming her to my little apartment to spend nights. We came to throw about that "L" word awfully fast. The euphoria wasn't to last.

One evening, when we were together, Sharon's husband started to ring my phone. She told me not to answer. This was in the stone age of phones, when they were tethered to the wall with wires. The husband did not stop. He left hysterical messages, replete with the possibility of violence. After a few progressions of this, I took the phone line out of the jack, but all that did was substitute my imagination for the menace of his voice. When Sharon left for work in the morning, I picked up the telephone and had a conversation with the man. I was prepared to let him know that I had a loaded Winchester rifle in the house, but my talk alone seemed to be calming him down. We ended the conversation, I propped the unloaded rifle in a corner, and I did not hear from him again.

A day or two slipped by with no contact from either of them. I wound up into a coiled spring. The soles of my feet started an annoying painful spasm I sometimes get. I would get out of bed sneezing from spring allergies, my eyes watering, my chest tight. I drove to the shore just to get some air. I hit the nearest commercial strip and got a submarine sandwich I could not finish—not because it was too large but because the bread had neither texture nor taste. I stopped at a seafood shack and had some greasy fried shrimp. Food was not cooperating with me, increasing my cravings rather than satisfying them. I waited out the cravings, coming to a point where I forgot about hunger entirely. I could not bring myself to pick up the now poisoned telephone. I could not even touch it.

A few days later, Sharon appeared at my door. "You played right into his hands," she screamed. "I only came here to get my things."

"How did I play into his hands?"

"*You* know."

"I don't know," I said. I did not know.

Sharon extracted her t-shirt, hair dryer, a book and two audio CDs and stormed out without saying anything else. My brain swirled with pollen. She wants me to follow her, but I cannot breathe. I have a few moments to redeem this situation, before she starts up her car, but let her go—I can find another girlfriend—they are easy to find—but one who is not wacko!—My moment evaporated. I trailed around the yard, having an idea that I would calm myself by taking in the full of green spring. Pollen shrouded my car, and I could feel the stuff seeping into me through my nasal passages and even my eyes. I came back into the apartment, showered, holding onto the heat from the water in an attempt to open up my breathing. As the water thundered over my head, I tried to run the fatal telephone conversation in my mind, but I could not latch onto it. Should I have mentioned the Winchester? Should I even have a firearm? Wasn't there some kind of Connecticut firearm registration law? Paperwork I haven't done? A check I needed to write? There has to be, in this state that veritably drips with laws—they even levy *a property tax* on your car, not a sales tax (which they also have), not a vehicle registration fee (which, of course, they have), but a tax *on the assessed value of your vehicle*. I did not know then but know now that obsessive attention to detail like this is one of anxiety's great calling cards. Days-full of detail seemed to follow one another. I do not rightly know how many of them elapsed. Two? Twelve?

The detail ground into rubble, then cinders, then powder. My brain could not latch onto anything. I circled the room, hoping fatigue might wind me down. I recall trying to write, attempting to revise a draft of a book I had just written, but the well was dusty and dry. Nothing came out when I sat down at my computer. I have never suffered from writer's block, but this was not writer's block, it was paralysis, person block. I hunched over the screen and read through what I had of the book, and decided it was pretentious trash. I kept it, but took my name off the title page. If I died without being able to arrange my affairs, I did not want a strange somebody or even a relative to know that I had anything to do with that awkward study of human achievement. Too many books are written on this tedious subject. I can sum them up in a few words: Get out there. Do. I would follow my own advice, but it would take some time.

I drove down to my parents' house. My father, already retired, was home, sitting in the living room in his worn gray tracksuit, reading the New York Times. I told the man I was suffering from uncontrollable anxiety. What was my purpose in doing this? Did I really expect advice? My father immediately went into a reverie, and described in detail the three times in his life that he had suffered from anxiety, as if I were bringing up the subject to allow him to expound on it from his own personal perspective. I listened, not out of politeness, but because there was no stopping him. I don't remember what the three occasions were, only that there were three. My mother attempted to feed me, but

in the state I was in, I could not risk being poisoned. I
played the piano I grew up with for a while, treated myself
to a bacon cheeseburger with fries at the local diner, and
then went back to my wife's house. I let myself in, and
waited the day until she came home from work. She took
me back.

I saw a doctor, and got on some anxiety medication. It did
not give instant relief, but it helped me take off the edge. I
still needed to do something, so I did something. I enrolled
in a full-time, professional cooking course. The fourteen
weeks was hard work. I was the oldest in the course by
twenty years, and the only male. I literally cooked my way
out of anxiety. I then had a job with a caterer, cake baking,
moved into food writing, took to that, won some awards,
and wrote a musical comedy along the way. The marriage
simmered for seven further years and finally boiled over for
good. I expected some anxiety, but instead I felt elated and
free. In taking stock of things after a few months of living
on my own, I looked back on the anxiety I had gone
through with Sharon. It seemed safely lodged in the past.
Experience would protect me in the future. I had no way of
knowing I was in for something far worse.

It took another woman. (This is my point of view—she
would tell the story differently, if you asked her.) I do not
seem to have any luck with women. Julia and I met online
and fell instantly in love. Within a year, we were sharing a
large house in a small town in rural Connecticut. Yes, the
anxiety state. (I ought to stay away from Connecticut, and
generally do, except when I go up to New Haven to
participate in a Parkinson's research project.) When you
have a relationship with someone, you need to ask yourself
honestly how many people are actually involved. In the
first Connecticut disaster, ten years before, the answer had
been four: the two of us, her husband, and my wife. In the

second case, three entities were involved: the two of us, and alcohol. The mix was volatile. I was commuting to wine school at Johnson and Wales University in Providence, Rhode Island, soaking up far greater levels of knowledge and perspective than I was ingesting alcohol. I studied, haunted wine shops, tasted, made my notes, read widely, and took an exam for my first wine certification. For me, alcohol was a segment of human civilization, for the woman, it was a chemical, a reverberation of family pain and parental abuse.

When I met Julia, I had recently been divorced, but I had had the opportunity to try to stand back from my experience. I had briefly seen a counselor with the aim of improving the choices I had been making. I created an extensive journal on the subject, identifying several personality types that had burned me in the past—anger, chronic depression, self-entitlement, unavailability. I certainly had my own problems and quirks. I was undoubtedly Mister Wrong for many a woman, but that is subject for another book (and I am not going to write it). As an aware person, I thought I knew about alcoholism, but later I was to realize that I had never before encountered the visceral and altogether horrifying face of it among my family, friends, or in any of my relationships. I already had a James Beard Foundation Journalism Award nomination for my writing in the beer wine and spirits category. If someone had asked me then if I knew about alcohol abuse, I would have answered certainly, yes. I did not know what I was talking about. I learned the hard way, and I nearly lost my life in the process.

Alcoholics, like the beverages they abuse, come in a number of packages. I was faced with the species *alcoholatis manipulatis*. In speaking years later to others who have had front line experience with alcoholics, my description usually leads them to nod grimly. Manipulative alcoholic children inherit their manipulative alcoholism from manipulative alcoholic parents. Julia gave me a thorough tutorial in alcoholic dysfunction. She did not attack me straight out. She did her research first. I was the subject, and she was the expert. She knew how to talk to me, how to coax me instantly into bed, how to destroy my equilibrium and balance, and ultimately just how and where to dig her nails into me and cut into my persona. You get sucked in, your good will used against you.

After we had a denouement, in a brief moment of apology, she admitted that she had been mirroring the dynamic she had grown up with, her mother's ceaseless persecution of her father over his chronic health issues. Before Parkinson's—at least I think that I did not yet suffer from the disease—my major health concerns involved difficulty breathing and allergic skin reactions. As things deteriorated between us, I came down with hives all over my body. As far as Julia was concerned, it was all in my imagination. Believe me—you know when your skin is crawling off. You know when you cannot breathe because oxygen does not get to the places it is supposed to go. If you imagine anything, it is the hopeful notion that you can find some way to breathe, so you can take this basic need for granted and get on with all the other projects on your plate.

Assuming that I in fact had a touch of hypochondria, James Parkinson himself (in *Medical Admonitions to Families*, 1801) wrote some pithy words about the phenomenon:

> "Such persons are particularly attentive to the state of their own health, to even the smallest change of feeling in their bodies; and from any unusual feeling, perhaps of the slightest kind, they apprehend great danger, and even death itself… The

strange capriciousness of their complaints induce
those around them to suspect them all to be
imaginary. This is, however, very far from being the
case. It is true, indeed, that from the constant
attention they are disposed to pay to every trifling
change which arises in their bodies, and from the
apprehensions with which they are tormented, their
account of their feelings may be rather exaggerated
and hyperbolical. But allowing this to be the fact,
and even that the most ridiculous and chimerical
distresses are imagined by them; even in that case,
their sufferings are such, that no considerate person
will regard them in any other point of view, than as
demanding all the solace and relief that friendship,
attention, and judgment, can bestow."

I do not recall receiving any solace or relief, just criticism
and "I know better."

> "I cannot quit this subject," wrote Parkinson,
> "without again noticing the folly, nay cruelty, of
> considering this complaint as dependent on the will
> of the sufferer; and remarking, that so far from this
> being the case, this disease particularly depends on
> the original temperament of body. As well,
> therefore, may the peculiar state of the patient be
> ascribed to him as a crime, as the distressing
> feelings he experiences be attributed to his caprice."

I might have had an early touch of Parkinson's disease at
the time, but I certainly did not have the benefit of the good
doctor's perspective and compassion.

There came a time when Julia started to travel a great deal
for her work. The hard edge of winter bit into me while she
was gone. I came down with a bad cold, desperate for

breath, took too much Sudafed, and ended up in the local emergency room with my heart beating a hundred and fifty times a minute. When the woman came home a few days later, she scolded me. "If I had been there, you would never have needed to go to the emergency room in the first place." This damaged shell of a human who could not keep her lips away from a bottle was lecturing me on emotional health. She kept travelling, leaving me in the care of my anxiety. The terror mounted and grew, like a piece by Tchaikovsky, constantly promising to come to a cadence only to move on to further themes and variations. Alone in that big house once again, nearly snowed in, spinning with self-generating fright, I held the barrel of my lever action Winchester to my head, trying to gauge whether my arms were too short for me to handle the trigger. I could just about make it, if my hands did not shake. They did shake. I decided to try again, when my hands were a little steadier. A shot of tequila might do it. If I squeezed the trigger steadily the way you are supposed to…

…A flash of logic shook me, even amused me. If I could figure out how to shoot myself without botching the job, I could figure out how to survive. That is, if I did not have an accident. If you own a firearm, and you have ammunition for it, in a moment of delusion you could misuse the weapon in any of a number of ways. I looked out the window at the winter sky. Daylight was fleeing quickly. I suddenly had an insight. I couldn't bring myself to throw my Winchester into the Connecticut River, which was just down the street from the house. If I disposed of the gun in some legal way it would take time, paperwork, but a gun without ammunition…that's a thought. There is nothing quite like having a mission. I drove several towns away and furtively threw all the cartridges into a dumpster. As I was driving back to the house from this horrifying transaction, I knew I had turned some kind of cathartic corner. I treated

myself to a large pizza, and stuffed myself into a calm I had
not felt in weeks.

Once I processed the pizza, further action became possible.
I called a family friend, a psychiatrist. He prescribed
medication, but warned me it would take some weeks to
work. It took its sweet time, but he guided me through it.
The medication began to tell. Julia criticized the
medication, saying it was changing my personality.
Obviously, she would have had a better solution. She gave
me that look—come to bed—but I resisted her. I did not
want her opinion. Selective insights may approach wisdom,
unedited spasmodic word torrents yield little.

She travelled again, I handled the solitude, enjoyed some of
it. We spent time together, going through the routine,
speaking little. My head began to clear. I came home from
a day trip to Manhattan one evening. She read something in
my manner. I had business to clear up on my computer
upstairs, I wanted to think about things, but she forced the
issue, threw a chair against the wall, and stormed out of the
house with a suitcase. A few days later, I got a vitriolic e-
mail from her. This led to a period during which we stayed
out of each other's way for several months. I would stay at
the house when she was away, and I arranged some wine-
related travel to Europe and California when she was home.
She sent me a conciliatory e-mail eventually. We shared the
house several more months after that, but I refused to sleep
with her, although she pulled out all the seductive stops. I
know when something is bad for me. The late spring
afternoon we finally liquidated the house, she told me she
loved me. I said nothing. It was the cruelest statement I had
ever made, but she gave me the chance, and I seized it.

I spent three years on the medication, tapering off ever so gradually. I moved back to New Mexico, started climbing in the mountains, and finally sold the Winchester.

Some years later, still in Albuquerque, I had the emergency room episode—that was month seven—in which my entire left side collapsed into weakness and trembling. This coincided with the full of the tree allergy season in the area. The inability to breathe I have had in June and July in Albuquerque was far worse than anything I had ever endured in the east. People have an erroneous idea that the desert is some kind of lifeless wasteland, but when juniper trees and sage bushes send their pollen into the air, allergy and asthma practices start to mint money.

I didn't know it at the time, of course, but I already had Parkinson's disease. Breathing issues are on the Parkinson's list. Dopamine deficiency causes the core trunk muscles that control inflation and deflation of the lungs to stiffen up. The ribs and lungs become cramped. Breathing turns into work instead of being an automatic think-nothing-of-it activity.

Desperate for breath, I moved back east. Arranging the move took a solid month, a miserable month. I could say I was unhappy, in discomfort and pain, but this was just my body reacting poorly to the environment—I was not having to deal with the uncertainty of a neurotic woman. As Bob Marley sings, "No woman, no cry." Having endured the two pervasive anxiety episodes, I had developed psychic antibodies—call it armor, call it scar tissue, call it valuable experience. Nervousness and uncertainty would certainly plague me for many months as I struggled for a diagnosis and appropriate treatment, but I never approached the cascading anxiety I had known in the past.

Ultimately, I was to realize that Parkinson's was my live-in partner. I shake when I get nervous, and get nervous when I shake, but this is not the hell of anxiety as I lived it. Part of surviving that was the certainty that I could never wind myself up that much again. Unlike another human, a disease has only the personality you decide to give it. The only human you need to factor into the equation is yourself.

Keep with me, for more on my brain (at risk) this time.

There is nothing either good or bad, but thinking makes it so—Shakespeare - Hamlet

Brain At Risk...The First Time Around

I was very young, and did not realize the brain was so important

I cannot be sure that I damaged my brain when I was a teenager, but I certainly gave it some stress (or exercise, depending on how you choose to look at it). I have asked a number of physicians whether psychotropic drugs can be precursors of or triggers for Parkinson's disease. They all answer that there is no known connection, but maybe all this means is that the relevant statistical research is yet to be done. If your brain goes to strange places at some time in your life, it seems to me that you have already crossed a certain reality boundary—permanently.

I am not always sure if I am experiencing reality. The other day, I was having a lie-down on my couch. I felt a sick feeling in my stomach. I got up, and retched into a paper supermarket sack I keep for desk trash because I did not have time to get to the bathroom. A minute or so later, I had to vomit in the bag again. I eased back onto the couch, hoping I was not coming down with another one of those two-week stomach viruses.

I do not want to get too disgusting in talking about this, but later when I took a look at the bag, it contained the usual wrappers and spent facial tissues. There was not the slightest sign of any vomit, nor did the bag have that characteristic smell. Parkinson's does compromise the sense of smell, which might give me difficulties if you were to ask me to analyze a 1959 Chateau Lafite Rothschild (this is a wine, and it costs five thousand dollars a bottle), but you would think I could still discern the presence or absence of vomit. My stomach felt fine, with not even the slightest queasiness. Could I have imagined the whole thing? My memory of the episode seems real enough. If I did imagine it, why that? It is clear that I "experienced" something that was at least theoretically possible. You could feel sick and retch into an upright bag. It is not as if [place your idea of a sexy female movie star here] had suddenly materialized in my apartment and I was unbuttoning her sweater.

And so, I begin to question which activities in the routine realm of the possible life are actually real—insofar as they are routine and prosaic, the imagination could inject them into my brain without suspicion or rigorous reality analysis. Most people think of Parkinson's as only a movement disorder, but the disease has an array of non-motor symptoms. The unpleasant term for this is "Parkinson's disease psychosis." The sufferer can see, hear or experience things that do not actually occur (hallucinations), or believe things that are not true (delusions). As with most aspects of the disease, "they" are not sure what causes the psychosis—it could be a side effect of dopamine therapy, an effect of the underlying disease, or both.

When you need to take pills multiple times a day, you encounter problems that at first seem to relate to memory, but ultimately they have to do with reality. It is not that you forget to take your dose, but rather that you cannot be sure you did not invent the dose-taking event. I cannot afford to rely on my memory/sense of reality in this regard. I set timers, and I use pill dispensers. I can reach back into my formative years and know that I invented reality. Once you invent even a scant morsel of reality and you process the event, you know it could happen again. Your cogitational innocence is damaged, your ability to filter reality crippled.

When I was a teenager in the nineteen sixties, I never read those books you were supposed to rave over, like *The*

Catcher in the Rye, and *Stranger in a Strange Land*. My go-to read was instead *The Pharmacological Basis of Therapeutics*, an encyclopedic guide to what drugs do that physicians used before the Internet. I grew up in a doctor's home. My father would bring home samples given him by drug company reps, and keep them in a drawer in the linen closet, right in the hall. The book told me the difference between those pills that were simply bad for me, and those others that could actually kill me. I was primarily interested in the amphetamines, what were then popularly called "diet pills" ("uppers" in the drug world). I might try an occasional sedative ("downer") just to see what it would do, but stimulants were my main squeeze, and the supply was virtually unlimited.

The drugs came with attached literature. I knew exactly what I was taking. There were other drugs I would get from people I knew—friends, their friends, and their friends—for which this was not the case. Marijuana was always wafting about. Then there was LSD—lysergic acid diethylamide, which I and all my contemporaries resorted to liberally. There is much misinformation broadcast about "acid," specifically that it causes hallucinations. This is not so, or at least it was not so in my case. When you have a hallucination, what you see is real. You might later realize it was a hallucination, but when it occurs it is as real as an IRS audit notice. In my case, no matter the level of pulsating kaleidoscopic perception I encountered, I at all times knew I was being affected by a drug.

Back in those days there was a major rock band called the Moby Grape who came out with an evocative song called *Hey Grandma*: "Robitussin makes me feel so fine/Robitussin and Elderberry wine." I used to favor Vick's Formula 44 cough medicine. The active chemical is called dextromethorphan. This is related to today's street drug PCP. At its proper dosage, the medicine is designed to work on what the commercials used to call the "cough control center" to ease you out of the spasmodic coughing cycle. Guzzle a bottle of the stuff all at once, and the cough control center dedicates itself to other pursuits, as one web site puts it, "It may produce distortions of the visual field - feelings of dissociation, distorted bodily perception, and excitement, as well as a loss of sense of time." Remember, I was an educated drug user. I knew what this drug did that even LSD could not. This drug melted the barrier between distortion and reality—what you imagine, you experience. You do not just *receive* random hallucinatory messaging— you *live* a different existence. Later, if you are introspective, you realize what happened. Reality is never the same again.

In medieval times and before, deadly nightshade (belladonna), mandrake, jimson weed and other substances that have similar effects to the cough medicine were used in witchcraft to melt that barrier between distortion and reality. Users did not think they walked through walls or flew on broomsticks, they knew they did. These drugs are "deliriants, which lead to a heightened sense of awareness and experience, as opposed to "psychedelics." which lead to heightened lucidity and perception. LSD bends reality, while the deliriants bypass it. The reality of 1968 was worth putting on hold, even if briefly. I do not mention opiates. I tried opium and heroin, one time each, but this apparently was not what I was looking for. Much later, in the 1980s, cocaine was coming into vogue, and my set of friends often passed it around. I enjoyed it immensely, but if the supply ran dry, I did not go out and try to find any.

Closer to now, a drug I do sometimes still take acts on that reality bridge. You have heard of it—it is called Ambien, Zolpidem, it is a sleep medicine, and it has an evil side. If

you take Ambien, first make sure your car is parked, your
door is locked, you are off-line, and your phone is
somewhere out of reach. Put your PJs on and floss and
brush your teeth before you take the pill. Dental floss
accidents are never pretty. It is possible to do things and
say things under the influence of Ambien and have no
recollection of the event. I have done this. I once
proclaimed my undying love to a woman for forty-eight
minutes over the phone. To another woman, in person, I
have reason to believe that I confessed my every sexual
thought and fantasy—all of it—you know, the odd and
convoluted things that you generally keep to yourself—you
have got your own and I do not want to know. I have been
to the all-night supermarket, and have found packaging
from which food has been untimely ripped in the car the
next day. When I take Ambien, I am rarely alone. I hear
people talking in the other room. I cannot tell the gender of
the people or the language they are speaking. I go take a
look just to be sure, but when I get back to my chair I can
still hear them. They have a benevolence about them, but I
am always aware their good intentions could evaporate. I
do not want to know them *that* well. Oh, what is that?
They're opening a 1959 Chateau Lafite Rothschild? Just for
me?

A key rule applies when your brain leaves your body to slip
into the next room in order to taste a legendary wine—you
do not get to keep the empty bottle as proof (but neither do
you get the bill). It's a fair enough trade.

I keep my Ambien downstairs and around the back of the
building, locked in my car.

It is impossible to know if any of the drugs I have taken
over the course of my life have done damage to my brain or
contributed to my Parkinson's disease. My main treating

physician tells me no. I did start with the *leucine-rich repeat kinase 2 (LRRK2)* gene, but the disease also needs a trigger, and the experts admit they know little about triggers. The easy inference in the case of Muhammad Ali, as one example, is head damage from boxing, but Ali's family believes his Parkinson's trigger was actually pesticide exposure suffered at a training camp in rural Pennsylvania. My own boxing career consists of hitting a bag, which doesn't hit back, but as to pesticides and chemicals in the environment, aren't we all somewhat vulnerable? Far from having a certainty in this department, I don't even have a palpable maybe. The math tells me that I have had a lifetime of exposure to environmental chemicals, compared to scant exposure to psychotropic drugs.

Even if drugs have not affected my brain, however, they certainly have affected my mind, what I do with my brain. They have affected my relation with reality. We are not talking here of an inability to "face" reality, which would qualify as a psychological or emotional problem, but of an expanded definition of reality that has the ability to bring in the good as well as the bad. Of course, I am looking out for the good it might do me. We writers hold on to any bit of imagination we can find. At the least, if I ever do suffer from "Parkinson's disease psychosis," a part of me will recognize what is happening, assuming I get the chance to look back on it during lucid moments. My radar is up for it. So far, scant if any blips. Other than the "missing vomit" incident, I cannot think of a time during my Parkinson's years when I have had a clear sensation of a hallucinatory or delusional event, but once bitten, twice shy. I can emotionally handle the reality of having a serious disease, you bet, and an occasional mind game might even be fun (I can write about it), but if I lose touch with reality consistently and repeatedly, I am going to be very scared.

Remember, when I was young, I took drugs to get there. Without drugs, I did not get there. I had a choice. Now, I am not so sure.

I read plenty often of notions that we all live in a computer simulation—we are all some variation of algorithm in an informational big bang. As artificial intelligence doubles and redoubles on itself, it must affect our intuition of reality, at least causing us to be highly philosophical about that which we call real. Reality requires more than simple evidence. It requires value. It requires relevance. It requires context. I do not know about your brain, but my brain both interprets and creates reality. Out of respect for this phenomenon, combined with an abiding fear of it, I cross the street with the greatest of care, knowing that my brain could "decide" the coast is clear only to be proved terribly wrong. It is not enough that I determine that no cars are coming—I want the additional protection of a "walk" signal. If the walk signal seems a little stale, I am willing to wait an extra ninety seconds until I get it afresh. I owe my three grandchildren at least this level of care.

When I go to a toy store with my grandchildren, I keep each kid to a strict five hundred dollar limit.

Grandchildren

It all depends on genes, as long as the bad one doesn't get through.

I am primarily of Ashkenazi Jewish ancestry. Some of us carry and may transmit the *leucine-rich repeat kinase 2 (LRRK2)* gene. If you have the gene, you are more likely to come down with Parkinson's disease. I have it, and two of my sisters have tested positive for it. When I first went out into the world, long before I knew about LRRK2, I made efforts to expand the gene pool. I married a Danish woman (in Denmark), and we gave our son and only child a Norse name: Thor Bjarke Essman. Thor's mother and I divorced when he was four. Thor married an Australian woman, Joan, whose family is from the Philippines. He has been living in Australia since 2002. Thor and Joan have three children, my granddaughter Selena, born in 2008, my grandson Lenox, born in 2010, and grandson Felix, born in 2014. Because Thor's mother and I raised him to have some connection to his Danish heritage, the Danish terms "Farmor" (father's mother) and "Farfar" (father's father) survive to describe us as grandparents.

I have twelve trips to Australia under my belt. The flight from Los Angeles to Melbourne is fourteen hours. The plane leaves LAX around 11:00 pm, already 2am according to my New York body time. If you leave on a Tuesday, because of the International Date Line, you arrive on a Thursday—Wednesday disappears somewhere over the Pacific. You also cross the equator, meaning that April becomes the equivalent of October. Spring into autumn is not so bad, but I have also done summer into winter and winter into summer. This is a good way to come down with a nasty cold or bronchitis.

I live in an English-speaking city, I fly over the largest ocean on the planet, pass over exotic places like Fiji, Tonga and Tahiti, and then arrive in another English-speaking city. Admittedly, their town has a well-managed beach where my town has a stretch of sorry sand, but my town has better Mexican restaurants. Much better. There is no outback or crocodile hunting involved here, just suburbia. Instead of getting my grandchildren Chinese toys at *my* local Toys-R-Us and hauling the toys to the other side of the world, I buy the same Chinese toys for them at *their* local Toys-R-Us. Afterwards it might be a trip to McDonalds or perhaps an expedition to Costco.

The two countries are not identical of course, but compare them to any of the hundreds of other countries on the planet, and they are close cousins. You do have to remember to look the other way when you cross the street. And—oh yes—we talk funny.

My annual Australia trips punctuate my life. I usually stay for about two weeks. I took my seventh trip, when I was just a few months into the illness sequence. I did not then perceive much was wrong with me, except for pulsating pains in my leg. I had energy, and everything went well. My son and I worked out together at the gym, I took long walks, and I energetically stood by the kids (at that time, just Selena and Lenox) at playgrounds and swimming lessons.

My eighth trip was something else altogether. I had as yet no diagnosis, no treatment. When you travel like this and you feel drained of energy, jet lag is the usual suspect, but I had faced and overcome jet lag seven times before—this time it seemed to be winning. I forced myself to do the usual activities with the kids. Watching the many hours of cartoons in the TV room was not strenuous. I bring eight puppets with me each trip—I think over the two weeks I managed to put on a single puppet show for the kids. I bought them toys of course, and ice cream, and pizza. I sat with Joan and the kids for the Easter service. The Philippine connection led to the kids starting out in the world as Catholics. My son and I are both non-believers, but I am capable of sitting in a church and enjoying the smell of incense. Thor did not attend. I did not kneel at the church, but did later bend down and address my future grandson Felix, due to be born in two months, to give him my own indoctrination. I wanted to keep the talk short and to the point. "Yankees!" I wailed repeatedly at Joan's middle. I know I got through.

The day before I was to fly back, I walked back to the house from the beach with Thor, Selena, Lenox and their big poodle Loki, in a stooped shuffle I was later to recognize as typical of Parkinson's disease, dreading each exhausted step, wishing I had a cane, savoring every bench. I call this my "exhaustion march." I knew by the time I slid down onto my bed and closed my eyes still in my shoes that I would have to see a doctor as soon as I got over the return-trip jet lag, if ever I did. I had great trepidations about getting the proper care—it would in fact take me nearly two years to get it—but I had to start somewhere.

Felix came into the world the day before I sat with my sister Nora at a neurologist's office and got the erroneous MS diagnosis. I thought of the three kids and wished I could assure them I would not fail them. To be there for them and yet…to be physically limited when they need me. The prospect was wrenching. We only get each other for two weeks. They expect and need energy from me. They are not blind—they can tell Farfar is not doing that well. When Nora dropped me back home, I ordered my new medication and vowed I would use it over the next ten months to somehow, some way, bring myself to the energy level they expected of me. I was later to learn that Copaxone prevents the MS from getting worse, rather than make you feel any better. It is no help for Parkinson's, completely useless. I had the MS diet, of course, and I was pinning high hopes on that.

The months to come consisted of jabbing myself daily with MS medication, stuffing myself with line-caught salmon and kale, doing everything I could to keep my head above water, always with the three precious ones on my mind. My "Grand-Kids" folder swelled with shots and short videos of Felix, and yes, he often wore his tiny Yankee cap.

The year turned and my ninth trip was booked. I was making careful plans as to how I was to assure a sufficient supply of individual-dose Copaxone syringes for the trip—these have to be kept cold. Unlike normal drugs, Copaxone had to be shipped in dry ice from a special pharmacy with a tight window between shipments—you are down to only a few day's supply when the next shipment comes in. I figured I would fly a week after a shipment, meaning I should be nicely back home by the time the next shipment arrived. I worked it all out, but then I would also have to arrange to keep the drugs in the family's refrigerator in some way that the kids would not mess with them, or even know they existed.

While still enmeshed in this sequence, I switched doctors, switched diseases, and switched drugs (two months before my flight). The new drug was not doing much—I would not know for many months that I was being under-dosed, but the drug was generic and I no longer had supply concerns. My only calculations were how I was going to handle the two older kids with an energetic ten-month-old added to the mix.

Australia trip nine was an absolute disaster. I do not mind writing this because Australia trip ten, which occurred after my health improved, went exceptionally well. I remember one joyous thing about trip nine, throughout the two weeks: Felix straining to stand up on his own, nearly making it, falling, trying again to imitate his big brother and sister, pushing himself to the limit to succeed. I watched and knew I would miss those first steps, but not by much. I missed my son's first steps—he was in Denmark at the time. The rest of the trip is a blur of struggle. On the second day, I attended Easter service again. The priest had chocolates and kind words for all the kids. I dragged myself around, slumped into a folding chair in the park afterwards as the kids and all their friends searched for Easter eggs. Serious picnic accessories and furniture appeared. Everybody wanted to meet Thor's dad. I made conversation as well as I could. At one point, a young boy came up to me shyly and turned back to his mother asking, "Who is that strange old man who doesn't speak?" I could not strategize my way into words, but I wanted to say, "Haven't you ever heard of baby boomers, Kid? We're never supposed to get old." Old is what I felt, but I was not so distressed that I could not see a strange bit of Easter irony—all these bunnies and candies, balloons and streamers are bright pastel signs of spring, and yet here in the antipodes the blustering winds of winter are just around the corner. In this odd land where everything is upside down and in reverse, Santa Claus walks around in shorts.

I was better by trip ten, had energy. The only down note was that this time I forgot to bring the puppets. I was certainly ready to be well. Felix was by this time walking. I played light sabers with my three Jedi knights. Lenox woke me every morning and asked me to play the card game Uno with him. Selena would discover us and join the game. The kids took real delight in shouting out whenever I forgot to declare that I had only one Uno card left. I happily paid the two-card penalty. I attended their tennis lessons. We went to an adventure park. Knowing that my medication was finally appropriate, I was able to strategize the activities I did with the kids. I knew my limits, but I was determined to break through them, at least a little. I took it one day at a time, one hour at a time. When they conked out, I took a power nap. When I had an extensive jet lag conk, their mother gave my excuses and they even giggled at my snoring.

The need to concentrate my time with the kids brings both pressure and joy. If we lived near each other, we would enjoy quiet time together, all in little interspersed bits, in economical units of time. Situated as we are on opposite sides of the sphere, the time is so dear, so expensive, that every moment has to count. The other grandparents are reasonably close, in Sydney. I do not compete with them and yet I cringe at the math: they see the kids more often, in a more involving way. I am friends with them on social media—they frequently post photos of the kids. They are the Philippine "Nana" and "Nano" just as we are the Danish "Farmor" and "Farfar." Even though my grandchildren know who I am on some levels, on others we must get to know each other all over again on every trip. The other grandparents do not need to do this. They have continuity.

I cannot change the fact that it took years for me to get a handle on my health, but I am glad that during those years I did not skip the difficult trip once. I miss all three of them terribly now, but the day will come when we will be able to play light saber and even watch those inane cartoons together. I am looking into ways I can coax my son into having the test to see if he has that gene. In the meantime, I

sometimes take the puppets out and have a long strategic
talk with them. We rehearse routines. The year will pass
and we will be ready.

If you keep digging for value...

Some Things You Keep

I need to get this said here, now!

I need to say this thing here, now, before I cover any other issues. It surprises me. If I could take a pill or even have brain surgery and suddenly not have Parkinson's disease, I certainly would take advantage of the chance, but not right away. I would wait and hold on to the disease a little while longer, end my relationship with it gradually, let go one little piece at a time. I would have to say a proper good bye. Even if it were gone, I would make it clear that I would expect an e-mail from it now and then, a social media comment, and of course a keepsake. I know just the thing—collect whatever medication I haven't gotten around to using and have it all bronzed, frame it, and display it on my wall next to my diplomas.

Parkinson's colors my thinking, my seeing, my work and my planning. When I look back to the person I was before I had symptoms, before I had any uncertainty as to my physical condition, I get a fill-in-the-blank human being. I can, and do, write about that person, but I cannot emotionally relate to him. He is a stranger. The books he wrote are on my shelf, his family photos on my computer, his contacts list on my smart phone, his impressive social media network at my fingertips, but I look at him and realize I am just getting to know the man. He seems an intelligent sort, creative, but a flawed entity when it comes to his relationships.

Yes, I am just getting to know him. If he had not had Parkinson's disease, I would possibly be able to describe him, but I would not know him as well as I do now. He now sits at his computer with his shirt off, cooling off from a trip to the gym. It is snowing outside, the streets covered in fluffy white. He feels whole and complete, suffused with a sense of wellbeing, as he works on this book. He likes this feeling and wishes he could turn it on like a light. Maybe he can. Give it some time. Give it some time.

When you write something, especially something ambitious and sizeable, and you look back at it after a passage of time, and you change, you have to get to know the author all over again. Some of this process can be uncomfortable. Who did I think I was, writing that? Why did I choose to express myself in that way? Do I really want to leave my individuality open for anyone—totally out of my choosing—to pore over, without the slightest ability to answer for myself? I can answer that—absolutely, yes. There is power in vulnerability. If I succeed in bringing across my flaws, and I have so many, I establish in so doing my strengths, I should hope in equal degree.

I have had supreme moments of calmness and integrality during the writing of this book. These fine moments came to me only because I had a physical and mental challenge. I have had serious challenges at times during my life. Certainly, my periods of anxiety were important. I survived them as I have described, but experienced little in the way of growth. Survival, chugging along, putting one foot in front of the other, only goes so far. At some point, either you lift your wings and begin to fly or the earth swallows you up.

The disease has not gone away. In plain-as-day fact, I have it, and cannot give it up. I am pleased to be managing it so effectively. If a bad turn were to come, if the medication stopped working as well as it does, I would be able to handle it, go on with my work, adjust as I have to. My eyes see clearly now, when so often in the past I had to grope in the dark. I can tell you why in a single word—focus. We think we know what this word means, but it is a slippery word.

You have peak performance gurus out there who preach—rather tediously—that you need to focus. Just cut through the clutter and do it, they say. Many of them do not realize that the ability to focus is often an inborn skill, like the ability to carry a tune. Something in their background they might not even be able to touch distilled their once amorphous potential into focus. Early trauma can knock it into them. Actor Sir Laurence Olivier related how his mother's death when he was only twelve wrenched him out of childhood and into serious work in the theater. Olivier's grief served as a clear-cut catalyst. Adversity has a way of cutting through mists.

My own adversity—Parkinson's disease—gave me the first sustained focus I have ever enjoyed. I have had brief *moments* of focus—I do well on wine and spirits exams—but lasting long-term focus eluded me. You know the word, you may even be able to wax eloquently on the subject, but you cannot understand this thing unless you plug into it. Where and how you plug into it is the great issue. The bumps of life seem like a good place. You are not going to find the raw material of focus in the upscale neighborhoods.

For most of my life, I was out of focus. That's right—a blur. When you are out of focus, you send energy out in all directions in the hope that some of it will hit a target of value. You flail around ineffectively. You complete a task or two, and then you reach for the remote. I will not belabor this point—because now it applies to somebody else. I am very fond of myself, but I do not like that other guy very much. Parkinson's gave me a great barrier, but started to whisper to me I could break through. The process was not

instantaneous, but I kept hearing the whisper. The time
came when, without perceiving that I had gone through the
barrier, I stood on the other side. The disease is the same on
either side, but I am magnified many times. I cannot
quantify this change except to say that it is exponential. I
have reached into my integral self and discovered purpose
and value.

It is a great beauty of focus, once it infects you, that it
breeds further focus. Yes, I had my mission—write this
book, publish it, spread the word, make it a success. I had
that, but I did not have to restrict focus to the great projects.
I went to the gym this morning—focused. I cleaned the
snow off my car on my way back from the gym—focused. I
know it sounds like a cliché, the trite stuff of the
motivational speaker, but there is a reason focus is so
heavily extolled—it works. It is not a holy grail, always
beyond reach—it is something you can touch.

A Silver Lining

Despite the fact that peak performance and positive
thinking gurus and pundits have always nauseated me, I
have not ceased to look far and wide for some kind of silver
lining to my Parkinson's cloud. I did not find it but it found
me. I took an art course to "get out of the house." I have
always had musical and linguistic talent, but felt I could
never really "do" visual art. I started to paint landscapes in
oils, and astonished myself. After I finished one particular
landscape, I had a conversation with it in the privacy of my
apartment. Skeptical as I tended to be, the work was good.
In a few strokes that artist (I felt he was someone else, a
stranger to me), had been able to show movement in the
environment: mountains, rivers, forests, the sky. I
communed with this brilliance for an hour or more, pacing
around the room trying to get to the bottom of it all. "This

has to have something to do," I finally told myself, "with Parkinson's." A quick online search determined that I was going in the right direction with my insight: the dopamine replacement medication I took was the suspected catalyst:

"Dopamine is involved in several neurological systems," explains Prof. Rivka Inzelberg of Tel Aviv University's Sackler Faculty of Medicine. "Its main purpose is to aid in the transmission of motor commands, which is why a lack of dopamine in Parkinson's patients is associated with tremors and a difficulty in coordinating their movements."

"But it's also involved in the brain's "reward system"—the satisfaction or happiness we experience from an accomplishment. Dopamine and artistry have long been connected. It's possible that patients are expressing latent talents they never had the courage to demonstrate before, she suggests. Dopamine-inducing therapies are also connected to a loss of impulse control, and sometimes result in behaviors like excessive gambling or obsessional hobbies. An increase in artistic drive could be linked to this lowering of inhibitions, allowing patients to embrace their creativity. Some patients have even reported a connection between their artistic sensibilities and medication dose, noting that they feel they can create more freely when the dose is higher."

The prospect of becoming a successful visual artist has motivated me beyond all expectation. When my pills kick in, I pick up my brushes. I remain astonished at what I have been able to create. Cure me? Of course, by all means, the sooner the better, it is about time, for all of us. Take it away from me?—Now—wait a minute—not so fast! I can do without the Parkinson's shakes, but I want to keep the useful part that has been paying such a large portion of my emotional rent. It is up to me to hold on to this particular bump on the log of life. There are some things you keep.

Sleep—always an if.

The Question of Sleep

Always an issue, and then you've got to struggle your way into it all over again the next night...and the next.

An Ernest Hemingway quote caught my eye recently: "I love sleep. My life has the tendency to fall apart when I'm awake, you know?" I wholeheartedly concur. Sleep is no waste, but is rather, as the Dalai Lama once put it, "the best form of meditation." If only I could turn the sleeping state on at will, stay asleep, get enough sleep. The act ought to be simple: you put on your pajamas, turn off the cell phone, put in your night guard, extinguish the light, scrunch into a pillow, and then…

…the uncertainty begins. Is it going to work? Will my body allow my waking brain to take the time off it so desperately needs? Will I need chemical assistance? Will I fall asleep quickly and soundly only to awaken seventy-five minutes later? The question of sleep is a basket of uncertainties for me. I do not call it a question out of a desire to turn an elegant phrase. My sleep is always an if. This hypothetical quality was in effect before Parkinson's disease. It applies with even greater force now. Sleep disturbance is a recognized Parkinson's symptom. This includes the inability to fall asleep at night, the inability to stay asleep, and the annoying and sometimes unsafe tendency to fall asleep at odd times during the day.

I have good Parkinson's days and bad Parkinson's days. On a good day, I might have some trembling in my left arm and hand, some throbbing of my left leg. On a bad day, my entire body hurts. My back seizes up and I feel stooped even when I am lying down. In either case, I wind the day down with television: British cop shows, news, or food competitions. On my chair or on my couch my physical condition seems to be a crapshoot. I could spend hours in relative comfort, gradually attaining a useful sleepiness. I might just as easily squirm for hours, wringing muscle, bone, and nerve, sometimes helped a little by sleepiness, but often helpless. I understand and accept the idea that the way I feel physically has a psychological or emotional connection. If there were something I could do about it, I would spend more time on it. Wine in the evenings does tend to knit together body and mind, but sometimes it only agitates. Sooner or later, I get to a point by whatever means that sleep is worth a try.

"And so," as Samuel Pepys writes, "to bed." This is usually about ten pm, sometimes earlier. I look at my bed as the solution to a full day of body stress, but the practice does not always come in line with the theory. Before I was properly medicated, it used to be very difficult for me to adjust my position once I got into bed. Now I snuggle smoothly into my comforter. Sleep might come rapidly once I lie down, but I could also migrate into concentric circles of thought. Those thoughts could simply waft along, or they could combine and conspire into an organized thought attack. When this occurs, I never know the duration, whether the event will wind me up or exhaust me down. Half dreams might start to poke their way in. I am often in a reverie about taking a journey. Others observe me, judging without verbal comment. I go through a series of adventures, sometimes getting through and sometimes finding my way blocked. At some point, the observers fade and the destination evaporates. I sleep.

I have fallen asleep in one try, or in stages, with a drug or most usually on my own. Now I need to stay asleep. When I dream heavily, I often wake up with the sensation that I have slept a full night—I wish—only to realize once the blur clears that I am only ninety minutes gone. If I feel desperate that I will not get further sleep, I might think Ambien, but, of course, for a reason, my pills are downstairs in my car. My crossword puzzle books are good sleep inducers, but my body is too lazy to get out of bed to go find them. I give my comforter a try, snuggling into it with the hope of drifting off again. The brain might be resisting sleep during one of these episodes, but at least the sleep I have already accomplished frees my body from Parkinson's pulsations and pain in the meantime. One way or another, if I wake at eleven pm or midnight, I will get back to sleep, although I earnestly wish I did not have to go through the two-stage process. Once I see three am on the clock, I cringe in fear, knowing that this is likely it. My impulse is to hide my sleep behind a wall to shelter it against…well, I am sheltering one part of my brain from another, am I not?

I need seven hours of sleep per twenty-four hour cycle. If in my bed I get five or six, I am usually not sufficiently sleep oriented to grab the remainder—the sleep collection agency will let me be for a time and then start to dun me for the unpaid balance.

The process of my rising from the bed is a deliberate one. As I write this, my typical waking time is 3:30 am. 7:00 am will be my first of three pill doses. A timer I set the evening before is ticking down to remind me about the pills. I hit my computer's "on" button to get it started booting up, do the same with my phone. I then have only one thing on my mind: tea. I brew it fresh, from leaves, my ritual—I have never gotten the coffee habit. As my tea cools, I am invariably computing on or reading some electronic device, sometimes wasting time, more often at work. The timer reminds me to take the pills at seven. I quickly gulp them down and get back to work. The collection agency will soon chime in, I reach a computational saturation point, I doze off on the couch. I lose track of how long I escape from waking consciousness—it could be fifteen minutes, it could be forty-five. I slowly ease out of the bleariness, thankful for the sleep, but suddenly desperate to regain my lucidity. It surfaces begrudgingly.

I might at this point get an idea or two to slather onto my screen, but I have already been quite productive, and so start to orient myself to get to the gym. The hour is early by most people's standards. I need that extra time to rev up, if I want a quality, integral workout. If I feel I am not mentally ready, I might read for a bit. I get there—fortunately on foot. When I finish my exercise routine at the gym, I reward myself with a good lie-down and stretch on the mats. Flat on my back, recovering, I reach a state of equipoise, which sometimes entails a few minutes of sleep. Hey—I pay dues for this. Back in my apartment, late morning, I usually get right back to work, taking my second dose of pills at noon.

I do not consider my morning sleep sessions to be naps, but rather extensions of my nightly sleep. The dreams I dream are night dreams, existentially rich. Naps when they happen are afternoon affairs, always on the couch, never on the bed. Nap dreams are more like daydreams, often superficial. Since I do not decide to nap—naps just happen—I never think to turn off the phone. My mother had a sixth sense that let her know I was napping, so this was when she called me. She maintained a squadron of telephonic deputies cleverly disguised as people who call to congratulate me on winning a free cruise or vacation—she was awfully sneaky this way. "Was." She cannot bother me any more—the game is over. I have deleted her distinctive ring tone from my phone. The memory of that tone still makes me cringe. Yes…she's dead—technically.

I passed my driving test easily—the fourth time around

Driving

I really do not want to kill anyone, really.

Have you ever driven somewhere in your car, arrived, cut the engine, and then realized you had no memory of the driving event? Of course you have, and this has also happened to me. Experts call it unconscious driving, highway hypnosis, or white line fever. The conscious and unconscious minds concentrate on different things. The conscious mind thinks about changing your weekly lottery numbers, convincing your partner to cater to your sexual obsessions, tinkering with your grandmother's oatmeal cookie recipe, while the unconscious mind does the driving. If you have an accident or a cop stops you, the disparate minds might merge. They merge when, finally parked, you get the odd feeling that you drove without noticing it, and then they separate again for your next adventure. Happens to all of us.

As a Parkinson's driver, I do not have the luxury of unconscious driving. I cannot rely on any degree of automaticity. I am operating a machine that can easily turn into a killer. I cannot simply take it for a spin. I need to mentally checklist every event, every partial turn of the wheel and quantum of pressure on the accelerator and brake. Although I have been driving for half a century, now I need to drive as if I were again the learner. It is as if I have a driving instructor who sits by me and gives commands: "Come to a full stop" or "Put on your right signal" or "He has the right of way." The smoldering brain takes the cue and obeys. If I did not employ the instructor, I might have to rely on a brain that might simply *decide* that the light is green rather than react to the reality of the road. When you get the idea that your brain might just get it wrong, your imagination…no, forget your imagination…just see that you get it right!

Let us be clear about this. In most life circumstances, delusion is only detrimental if it persists. In a car, a split second of delusion could be fatal.

You might not think of it, but driving requires you to do a constant calculus relating to the size of objects (both moving and stationary), their changing distance, your speed, and the speed of other drivers. You also have to factor in your take on what other drivers see and hear. Parkinson's disease compromises much of my ability to coordinate in space, to perceive relative distance. I cannot count on my driving experience to come into play when needed—my automatic switch is off. When driving, I need to drill into the experience, stick my hands into it, rub it all over the steering wheel, otherwise it is lost to me.

When I drive, I need constantly to monitor whether or not I am keeping my lane. This used to be a matter of instinct, but my instinct has perished, and I need to think about my distance to cars and trucks, and then think again. Is this hunkering SUV coming toward me a threat? Can I clear this wide parked truck? Is that kid about to dash across the street? I brake early, and have begun to take local speed limits literally. A yellow light causes me to slow down rather than speed up. I do complete stops rather than rolling stops at stop signs. Distance, speed, my ability to act and react, all weigh heavily on me as I navigate my unwieldy machine.

Given the challenge to my coordination, I need to keep a firm hand on the steering wheel. This is difficult to do when my left hand is feeling feeble, is shaking, or both. My left hand does not grasp or even feel the wheel with the same confidence as the right. It sticks to the wheel with some friction rather than holding onto the wheel with any pressure. All the while, the right hand remains firm and strong. I naturally favor my strong right arm and hand. When I move the wheel to the left, the pushing right hand provides most of the strength, the left accompanies. The right hand pulls, the left follows, when I turn the wheel to the right. The utmost coordinating effort commands the hands to work as a unit, with my body straining in between. I have not had an accident since long before my Parkinson's disease diagnosis, but the possibility rides with me like a passenger.

My left side distraction also pertains to the left leg. I drive an automatic and hence depend only on my right foot for accelerator and brake. I push my superfluous left leg fully into its space, straightening it out as best as I can in an attempt to calm it. The leg often begins to ache and throb, often just as the left hand starts to act up. After a time in which I feel the left leg and left hand annoying me separately, they communicate with each other, coordinating their attack on my equilibrium, conspiring to make me lose control of the killer machine. I would not be able to continue driving under these conditions if I did not have that reliable driving instructor at hand. The instructor resides permanently in the cogitating segment of my brain. "Ease on the brake" or "Leave an extra car length" or "Even though it might seem beyond the scope of human possibility, obey the 20-mile-per-hour school zone speed limit." The instructor does not want to hear any excuses, at least until we have safely parked and he is paid.

The act of parking my car presents me with a particular set of problems as I configure space and time with the acceleration and braking functions of the car. Parallel parking is never a single attempt. I will park further away from my destination if in exchange I get a nice big easy space. Even face-in or diagonal parking sometimes requires multiple attempts because of my inability to guide the vehicle between the painted lines with appropriate space right, left, front or back. I check my car once I leave it. It is often askew, which is all right, as long as all four tires are within the lines. I cannot be troubled with how the thing looks.

In exiting the car, I am forced to operate the handle with my weak left hand and push the door open with my left elbow and arm. My goal is to get the driver door open as widely as the space allows, anchor both feet to the ground, and stand up. No matter how much I progress in retraining my balance, however, I nearly always reel as I try to stand up. Leftward movements can be problematic for me. I am faced with a choice. I can regain my balance by taking a few left-leading steps sideways down the edge of the car, and then move back to the door to close it. Alternatively, and most usually, I brace myself by grabbing the top edge of the door with my right hand and arm, reeling and adjusting my feet until I reach balance. I have never fallen when exiting, but I have never exited without at least the perception that I was about to fall flat on my face. No automaticity here—I must plan, think, act and assess. Even when I slam the car door shut, I have to be wary that I do not force myself into a typical Parkinson's backward lurch.

Although I keep my driving local, about once a month my car needs his feed. Self-service gasoline stations are very public places. I for one certainly do not want to hog a pump, knowing that waiting drivers might be gauging my transactional abilities with the eye of professional baseball scouts. I want to be seamless, anonymous, efficient. Call it paranoia, but at a service station I pump adrenaline as much as I pump gas. My door-braced exit from the car is smoother than when I am not under this pressure. The gas-cap unscrews with a deft motion. The wallet and credit card extract with an admirable glide. I punch in my zip code with precision, hit the appropriate octane button, push the nozzle into the gas-tank, and brace myself with it against the car as the pump fills the car and depletes my funds. Smooth as silk, I could say, except for the imperceptible (to others) reel as I extract the pump. This I cure by screwing the cap back on and feeling connection with the solidity of the car. In contrast to my operation of the vehicle, the fueling process is automatic, subconscious, blissfully efficient. Once I fire up the car, the driving instructor confiscates my remaining adrenaline, my car becomes a box on wheels, and I continue to concentrate on avoiding disaster, all effort for an errand.

*The fear of death follows from the fear of life. —
Mark Twain*

Mortality

Death is not listed on my current lease, but the day will come when it is the only tenant.

Death comes in many colors. My own death, as a concept, bothers me least, personally, but the prospect of it causes me distress for the sake of those I leave behind. You see, I am convinced that once I die the world will continue on its course. Young people will continue to grow until they run things, the music and wine I love will continue to spew forth, CNN will continue to latch onto news items and beat them to a quivering bloody pulp, all without my input.

I do matter, but the time will come—with my death and the passage of additional time—when I will not matter. If I were destined to be one of those physically ephemeral humans who etch their being and works on subsequent generations, a Churchill or Michelangelo for example, I would have gotten there already. I am a writer, of course, even an ambitious one, and there is some longevity inherent in that, but even that will fade. Some people love me, others like me, but these people will grow old and die in a cosmic instant, and the memories of me they carry will evaporate with them.

I speak of the grimness of death because it relates to the possibility of my own grim death, from as you read in obituaries "complications of Parkinson's disease," not inevitable but possible, wasting away, losing ability after ability, surviving to the point of human wreckage, beyond my darkest imagination. I have long figured that if I got a fatal cancer diagnosis like my father did I would skip the popular Elisabeth Kübler-Ross five step grieving process—denial, anger, bargaining, depression, and acceptance—in favor of an elegant two-step process: drug me into an

ecstatic stupor and then I die. If it takes me a generation to
wither and die of Parkinson's disease, I will live with death
to some degree every day as portions of me erode, the death
by a thousand cuts. I know this is rather a morbid way to
look at my possibilities, but I am not happy about this
dying process. I am philosophical, respectful of the beliefs
of others, but ultimately a non-believer. For me, death faces
me un-burnished, raw.

Death faced me without makeup, keen-eyed and all-
knowing, direct and to the point, on a January day, in the
Bronx, as my cousin Peter gave up and left us. We were
born only a few weeks apart (and now death is separating
us by years). The leukemia had promised us that it would
not take him, the care he received was supposed to be the
best, there was supposed to be more time, always more
time. All he wanted to do was get out to his boat, and all I
wanted to do was pick him up in Brooklyn and drive him
half the length of Long Island to get to the boat, that thing
he loved. It hardly mattered that neither of us had the
energy to make sail. For years, he had worked and saved,
ratcheting up previous boats for about the largest sailboat
he could possibly handle by himself, toiling at an office job
he hated. He finally retired, and soon after, he got a
diagnosis. The word seems sterile and tame: a diagnosis.
The body should do ones bidding—what temerity for it to
rebel, to etch into itself with sadistic self-hurt.

Peter decided to refuse treatment for a rare lung disorder
rather than live a compromised life. Because of debate as to
when and how we would drive my frail mother into
Manhattan to see Peter in the hospital, my sister Nora and I
kept delaying a final expedition. Parking was the issue.
Without my mother, it would have been simple—we would
have taken the train rather than driven. When Peter moved
to a hospice in the Bronx, I told Nora we had better make

the journey, not tomorrow—this evening, leave our mother out of it. Peter had just been admitted when we arrived. We had to wait half an hour before they would let us in to see him. The face masks and crinkly paper gowns they made us put on seemed ludicrous and unnecessary. What were we protecting him from if he was there only to die?

Harnessed with breathing tubes, Peter gyrated and struggled, jerking his body backwards and forwards, leftwards and rightwards. We announced ourselves several times, and bade him signal with a hand motion that he recognized us, which we later agreed he did. In his struggle—all was not peaceful—I couldn't decide if he was trying to live, trying to die, or stuck in some gray area in between. A moment soon came when Peter lay still, his head turned to one side. A nurse told us he was dead, but then she detected breathing. We left to collect our thoughts in the waiting area, debated whether we should get our mother, when we were summoned back and told by a young doctor that, "your cousin has passed away." Peter was an iconoclast and would have preferred the word "dead:" plop—the end—that's it—good bye. He should have left instructions as to the vocabulary. Nora burst into tears. My eyes were dry, but I could have used tears—the burning of what I saw still rages. I looked into the night as we left the hospice, then first realizing that the hospital where my son was born stood across the street—two ineradicable episodes of my life on the same block in the Bronx. I called my son in Australia to give him the news. I used the word "dead." We are not people who cannot face that thing.

We all met soon after to commemorate Peter. I wrote and recited this poem.

Even though we did not see each other that often

Whenever the opportunity arose
For you to make that barbed remark
I would hear it reverberating in my head
It still echoes
Bounces off empty edges
Soaks soft tissue
I have to imagine your remarks now
New input no longer
I have only to work with the past
The present speaks some other dialect
The future shrivels at my touch
I wanted to talk to you
Those last moments when you decided to
Go somewhere else
I had a premonition that evening
As I struggled to grasp the reality
Of the picture my mind had to paint
When Nora and I were with you those last moments
In the Bronx, deep in the Bronx
A place that means something
As we stood there paralyzed, mute, awash with pale death
You recognized us, you lifted your arms to show us that
you did
As busy as you were
As you struggled to live
As you struggled to die
As you took aim at something in between
Here are the words I left unsaid
To give you that final moment of balance
That ultimate sense that this is right
I bring you back so I can leave these words uttered
And so when we find ourselves together again
Whatever the mechanism
I do not know how it will happen but if there is certainty
I am as certain as I could be of anything
When we are together again

Somewhere, somehow, however we can explain it
Or even if we don't ever explain it
We will go out on your boat
With all the fuss that boats require
Seeing her shipshape and trim
Ready to heave anchor and cast off
The breeze will be tentative at first, but then
The sails will animate
We will reach open water
Pipe in some jazz, and finally share that joint

Peter's death left me—the word is as wrenching as it is
obvious—alive, and unaware of what I was supposed to do.
I want to say I wish I were not so grim, but I think there is
value in grimness, power in pessimism. I may be deep
within the grimness now, but remember that in this book I
have not remained a stranger to humor. I would not be
writing all this but to share. If I share my scorn at the slow
death I am experiencing I can better share my mirth and
hope. Grimness in proper context has value. I use it as I see
fit.

Shakespeare writes (in Henry VI, Part 1): "Just death, kind
umpire of men's miseries." I like the use of the word
umpire, an old French word that originally meant "odd
number, not even," hence a person who stands outside the
conflict, partial to neither side. Death is indeed just,
impartial, an equal opportunity employer, applicable to all
without exception, and it does erase our miseries,
permanently, or at least until the people we influence come
to mirror and magnify those miseries.

That mirroring and magnification are key, even if we apply
them to miseries, because we could just as easily attach
them to life's joys. Life goes on, even if we do not. Since
we are functioning portions of life, however small, we do

endure past our deaths. As our loss affects others, as they
shed their tears, and laugh at our never-to-be-repeated
jokes, as they curse us for our pigheadedness and
narcissism, as they commemorate us, as they damn and
revile us, we continue to live. If we write words—and I
do—we live. If we speak—and I do—we live. If we grab
each other in lustful excess, if we feed each other, if we
drink with each other, if we smile at each other, if we
scowl, if we scream at the top of our lungs in exasperation
at each other, even a stranger, we live. As many billions of
us are out there we, uniquely, live. I admit this is not grim,
not scornful, just a belief that I adopt as fact, otherwise
death wins, and death must not win.

Beer is made by men, wine by God." — *Martin Luther*

Wine on My Mind

I have actually written out wine prescriptions for my doctors. Somebody's got to help them channel their money in worthwhile directions.

I take the United States of America very seriously. The nation is not perfect I will admit, but I have a strong tendency to see it in its most hopeful light. Our nation has had a troubled relationship with alcohol, think prohibition, despite the fact that our founding fathers consumed astonishing quantities of inebriants. George Washington distilled and sold his own whiskey. Thomas Jefferson spent a fortune on wine. John Adams consumed huge quantities of hard cider and beer—often for breakfast. Alcoholic beverages were then considered to be safer than water, but beyond that, the founders needed alcohol to steel themselves for the tough business of winning our freedom and founding the republic. At the Boston Tea Party in 1773, what do you think the participants drank for courage: tea? They turned to their old standby rum to lubricate history, and they did not sip it demurely. Do you dare suggest that the convention in Philadelphia generated the Declaration of Independence under the chilly glare of sobriety? Stephen Hopkins, who suffered from Parkinson's disease, was not the only signer whose hand was shaking. Alcohol that day steadied many a quill.

In the musical film *1776*, Hopkins is portrayed as being over-fond of rum, demanding it constantly, but John Adams sets the record straight in his autobiography:

> "Governor Hopkins of Rhode Island, above seventy Years of Age kept us all alive…His Custom was to drink nothing all day nor till Eight O Clock, in the Evening, and then his Beveredge was Jamaica Spirit

and Water. It gave him Wit, Humour, Anecdotes, Science and Learning…And the flow of his Soul made all his reading our own…Hopkins never drank to excess, but all he drank was immediately not only converted into Wit, Sense, Knowledge and good humour, but inspired Us all with similar qualities."

Hopkins evidently knew how to and how not to use alcohol to lubricate social machinery.

Dr. James Parkinson himself, a near contemporary of the founding fathers, abstained from alcohol use, and in fact campaigned against its deleterious effect on the public health, condemning those who "spend a shilling on food and two shillings in the alehouse." Parkinson in his day was a political radical, took immense risks and was a steadfast supporter of our American struggle for liberty, and one can only imagine how he took the edge off. We ought to respect Dr. Parkinson's decision to shun the bottle, and ourselves avoid drunken excess—no need to swear off the stuff completely.

I began this book by stressing that, although I am rarely buzzed when you see me walking down the street, "I teeter and totter and might as well be drunk as a skunk." That is the Parkinson's disease. The question of my drinking is a thing apart, although alcohol for me does dovetail with the Parkinson's challenge. Like the founders (and unlike Dr. Parkinson himself), I too need alcohol to see myself through life's challenges. Then, as now, life without John Barleycorn, a metaphor for alcohol, is bleak.

I may have inherited the *LRRK2* Parkinson's gene, but fortunately I missed the gene for alcoholism. As I have discussed, I had a very painful romantic relationship with an alcoholic once. I hope never to go through that again. I am more of what I call a "reverse alcoholic," tending *not* to drink, falling far behind on my drinking. Visualize a late afternoon moment when I tell myself, "Go on, have a drink—it'll calm you down and even you out." Visualize a late-night moment of, "Drat—I forgot to have that drink and I really could have used it! Maybe tomorrow." That is about the size of it, a condition that might last for months on end. I am not aware of any support group for reverse alcoholics. Perhaps the people who campaign against drunk driving should add a plank against sober sitting. A breathalyzer test can cut potentially both ways. "You are not driving so why aren't you drinking?" Not in this country.

For most of my life, well into my fifties, I was wine blind. Given my lifelong interest in food and the good life, it is difficult for me to understand how I could have left wine in such a state of neglect for so long. Yet the unopened bottles, the unfinished glasses, the unlived evenings of convivial pleasure, stand as stark witness to the darkness I endured for a large part of my life.

It is astonishing, I know. I could drag in people who have known me in the past—kindergarten teachers, ex-wives, supermarket baggers—to testify as to my extreme sensitivity. Wine would seem to be right up my alley, but it is like the girl next door you do not notice for years and years. You leave home, you return for a visit, and there she is, a radiant beauty (and on the point of marrying some lout you did not like in high school). There stood wine, unrecognized and underappreciated.

My wine-blindness continued through my attendance at professional food school, my deep experience as a passionate "foodie," and my eventual involvement in food journalism and writing. When I was nominated for the James Beard Foundation Journalism Award for my newspaper food writing and someone at the awards banquet table mentioned she thought the wine was corked, I stupidly glared into my glass looking for specks of cork. I caught that look from the woman (she was too polite to correct me) felt sick in the pit of my stomach and realized that, yes, I had a knowledge gap to fill.

An online search that very evening nicely resolved the "corked" issue for me. A wine is considered "corked" and gives off a smell like wet cardboard if it is contaminated with a substance known as 2,4,6-trichloroanisole (TCA), which is usually the result of odd biological processes that occur, despite all efforts, in all too many corks. By contrast, a wine with bits of cork floating in it shows inept opening, nothing more. You need to strain the cork bits out but the wine is usually fine.

After the "corked" incident, my eyes began to open, and I began to see wine wherever I looked. Once I opened my first wine book and took my first wine course, once I sampled my first wine using a methodical tasting approach, I came to the realization that wine was the largest, most far-reaching subject I had ever encountered. I am an eclectic, a devotee of the liberal arts. Wine appears to be custom designed for *my* brain. It involves science, nature, history, geography, language, business, culture, law, government, interpersonal relations, sensuality and sense. Wine involves questions of taste. Wine is one of the binding forces in the civilized life.

That girl next door had finally managed to catch my eye, and I was in trouble. I became a wine and spirits writer, eventually earning both Certified Specialist of Wine and Certified Specialist of Spirits designations from the Society of Wine Educators. My background in wine certainly helps me approach my own drinking on a sophisticated level, but as I have already written, I also need alcohol to see myself through the challenges of my life, and that includes Parkinson's disease. The disease had diminished my ability to use the senses of smell and touch, but I can still feel when a wine is balanced, enjoyable, honest.

I enjoy drinking with relatives and friends, but also really relish a glass of wine or a shot of scotch or Tequila on my own. I might refill my glass if I am drinking with another person, but when I am on my own, one drink is the limit. I want to enhance my experience, not deaden my senses through drunkenness. Since I do not get around to pouring a drink every evening (I forget to do it—my reverse alcoholism rearing its ugly head), I probably account for about a bottle of wine a week. I do not want to argue this point with any reverse wine snobs out there, but life is either too short or too long to drink cheap wine. Good wine is expensive to produce. I do not mind paying twenty-five dollars or more for a week's wine if I get my money's worth. Cheaper wines almost invariably contain too much residual sugar, which I detest. These wines sell anyway because people like the way their labels look, or like the sugar, or both. There is no accounting for taste. Some people do not have any.

When I am feeling a particularly annoying level of trembling from Parkinson's and the drugs seem to be loafing rather than working, a moderate dose of alcohol neatly burnishes the physical edge, mollifies the mind, slowing down the ceaseless conveyor belt of time. This is not a result of the alcohol alone. The complex flavor components in a good wine also play a part. It is impossible to separate out the chemical effects of the flavor compounds from the aesthetic and sensory effects. When a wine is well balanced (balance is no empty catchword), the beneficial effects on the consumer of the wine reach a fine synergy. You do not miss the money. It is when you pay more and fail to get that evanescent balance that you look at your fingers and rue the fact that you now lack the cash to rub between them. You could have bought a thimbleful of beluga caviar with the same money, but you made your choice.

I revere many fine white wines. The two finest wines I ever tasted were a luscious Puligny-Montrachet and a flinty Chablis, both at the same wine show, both, oddly, pure Chardonnay. You spit into buckets at wine shows, and usually do not swallow, but even so, these two whites now have a permanent address in my brain. That said, the wines I usually buy and drink tend to be red. As I write this I am working on a French Crozes-Hermitage from the Rhône. The backup bottle is an Italian Barbera d'Alba from Piedmont. The Crozes-Hermitage is Syrah, and, since you are curious, I do favor that grape, from regions all over the world. At a higher Syrah level, I shared a 1999 Guigal Hermitage a while back with one of my ex-wives. We experienced a nice glow of togetherness with that one. A good Cabernet suits me on occasion and I do enjoy a Pinot Noir if it is extra fine. I consider Barbera my little secret, however. Barbera generates a delicious giggling high. At wine school, they do not teach you to evaluate inebriation levels, but I do.

Spirits in my repertoire consist largely of single-malt scotch and unaged Tequila or Mezcal. In either case, I drink these neat, with no ice and no mixers, at room temperature, the scotch with a little water to open it up. As with wine, I take a moment to appreciate the aroma of the beverage (as much as is possible given the inroads the disease has made on my sense of smell) before I allow it to slide down my throat.

The warming effect eases the Parkinson's trembling considerably. My brain soon feels the glow, my eyes begin to water, the lips tingle, my mouth fills with flavor, and I am either on a Scottish island or somewhere in the hills of Jalisco, depending on my beverage of choice for that month. The drink shunts the disease to one side for a short period, but if I did not suffer from Parkinson's I would have the same drink at the same time of day to evoke that glow the founding fathers enjoyed so.

The traditional English ballad "John Barleycorn" (and the song by the rock band Traffic of the same name) ends with a telling stanza:

> The huntsman he can't hunt the fox
> Nor so loudly to blow his horn
> And the tinker he can't mend kettle nor bowl
> Without a little barleycorn

Life without John Barleycorn is exceptionally bleak, and I am eternally thankful I discovered him, even if so late in life. He is of enormous help when I face the task of getting through a Parkinson's day. I will not over-drink to make up for the many decades lost to sobriety, but I am entitled to a measure of basic regret for all the healthy pre-Parkinson's time I wasted. The odd thing now is when I reel and stumble like a drunkard out on the street, once safely home I often turn to alcohol to coax my brain back to the middle. Alcohol well used is a fine thing.

I catalogue my entire experience of Parkinson's disease on this computer. It nicely edits out all the shakes.

Computing and Writing

I used to do this without thought. I now move constituent parts, fingers, wrists, hands as the chunks of my brain jangle and clink.

If I had an ordinary job—a chef, an auto mechanic, an Elvis impersonator—I would show up for work and do the job whether I felt like it or not. This option is not open to me as a writer. I certainly am able to plunk myself into a chair and tell myself it is writing time, but if I do not feel like composing, fingers do not strike the keyboard and words do not appear on the screen. Writing requires physical as well as cerebral effort. Since you are reading these words, you can guess that at least for a time this writer felt like it. What you cannot read is the dead time, the brain that refuses to engage, the back that rebels against the chair. In this very paragraph, you can interpret periods as stopping points not just for the reader but for the writer as well. Period: he stuffs his face when he is not hungry. Period: he goes for a pee when he does not really need one. Period: he checks his e-mail when he has just looked six minutes ago. The writer does not want it to be this way. He wants to be productive. He screams at his body and brain like a drill instructor, and is often hoarse when body and brain finally gel. The final output is the thing that counts, even if he gets it all done in poignantly small morsels.

Although as a professional writer I have keyed in literally millions of words, I never learned to touch type. For years, I might have been the fastest four-finger typist on the planet, but once the Parkinson's came into play, keyboard entry became arduous at best, impossible at worst. The problem lies in my left hand and fingers. I suffer the greatest level of Parkinson's trembling in my left hand, with added slight numbness. When I strike keys with my right fingers, I have the immediate sensation that I have completed a task. When I do so with my left fingers, I know cerebrally that I have entered a letter but can only be sure I have done it when the letter appears on the screen. I feel hand weakness as I type this sentence, and it is not pretty. Letters, as we know, have a way of becoming words, and it only takes a single error to interrupt my flow and put me into correction mode. Because my brain is involved, I make letter errors even when I write by hand. On a keyboard or by hand, I often begin words on the second letter, and then have to interrupt my thought process to correct the mistake.

I am right handed, but I can barely use a pen with that good hand. My writing hand has always cramped and ached after even a short effort. I slept through third grade and never learned cursive writing. My signature is all the script I can manage. At least I can read cursive, an important skill for a history junkie. Because it is so remote from my experience, I have come to admire fine penmanship. The Declaration of Independence, my first reference in this book, comes to us entirely in cursive. This is not the hand of Thomas Jefferson, its author, but that of professional calligraphers. Jefferson's handwriting was legible but not elegant. The president of Congress in 1776, John Hancock, set the standard, giving us what is certainly the most memorable signature in America's history, on the nation's very first day. The sloppiest signature on the document comes to us from the trembling hand of Stephen Hopkins. Like me, Hopkins likely suffered from a condition called dysgraphia, a profound interrupt in the ability to write by hand and another of the many aggravations associated with Parkinson's disease.

From my pen, you get a splotch of block letters, never effective, but now not even fully legible to its author. As I try to scribble with the right hand, the left one trembles and distracts. You need both hands to handwrite. The non-dominant hand is an important counterbalance. In my late twenties, I wrote an entire novel by hand. It is trash and I did not save the thing. I wrote some equally trashy fiction with a machine called, I think, a typewriter. You see it in old black and white movies. Made a clicking noise and poised professionals were experts in its use. Although I type with the wrong fingers, I got to be accurate and fast, but those mistakes I did make were always messy to fix. Word processing freed me from all the correction fluid, although not from the correcting process itself.

I use the left ring finger on my keyboard for the shift key even though, as I read, the pinky is preferred. My brain can only wrap around the left shift key—the right shift key is off my ergonomic radar. I do not always remember to hit the shift key. I constantly find myself recapitalizing letters. That left ring finger used to be extremely strong. I used it when playing electric lead guitar to bend strings. When trying to capitalize a letter, I often overcompensate by giving the left ring finger more push than it requires for shifting. I do no harm when I press shift with too much force, but when I miss the key and press "a" instead, I activate the repeat key function.

In these pages were once numerous instances of aaaaaaaaaaaaaaaaaaaaaaaa. I have, of course, ruthlessly expunged them all. All these extra aaaaaaaaaaaaaaaaaaaaaaaaa's would certainly thrill my doctor, but to this writer they represent just one of the many instances where I have to backtrack. I backtrack when I simply miss the letter key I want. I backtrack when my brain types a correct word but not the one I had in mind. It seems for every step forward, I take another step back. This might for a moment seem like a metaphor for my life, except that I edit my text. I am good at editing text but awful at editing my life.

The brain plays tricks when I compose text. Some are understandable, like typing in "stockings and blondes," when you mean to type "stocks and bonds," or "mutual fun" when you mean "mutual funds," or typing "send me a female" when you mean "send me an e-mail." Others are incomprehensible, like typing in "trout" when you mean "accessory." I might have absorbed this latter tendency from my most recent ex-wife (we communicate still). Monica would call women named Janet, Brenda, and call women named Brenda, Janet. I could not keep track and neither could she. My father years ago had a strange synapse in this regard. He appeared to declare that (singer) Andy Williams was "funny." It took a while for one of my sisters to figure out he was referring to then talk show host Merv Griffin. He confused Merv Griffin with actor Andy Griffith and then turned the Griffith into Williams. Then again, he would oddly confuse Purdue University with Tulane. He also confused other humans with objects of study, but that is another book.

I cannot guess what the bridge word between "trout" and "accessory" could be. Perhaps there are several. The human brain is supposed to be the most complicated machine in the universe, but it spits out the oddest output. We must expend enormous cerebral energy to come to these results. If only we could better focus. A good robot would not make these errors. When the robot malfunctioned, we could replace or repair a critical part, but this is not possible in the case of Parkinson's disease, which affects humans like me.

Every time I need to backtrack in my writing, I feel it literally in my back as I tense up. I put my back into my writing, and there is a cost. Every day, the back-endurance poker dealer up there allots me only so much back stamina. I usually get the annoyance in the middle or upper portion of my back, more a tightness and tiredness than a pain. I can sometimes renew my back energy if I get down on the floor and stretch out using my canvas stretching straps. Also, there come times when my brain becomes so content-rich that I type through every challenge. The back will then have to pay, but later. I take frequent breaks to lie down on my couch, often mindlessly turning on television news. Yes, more analysis, please! Once they drum the last vestige of the ability to think out of me, I move again to my computer, thirsty for verbiage, desperate for originality and determined to take care of that originality on my own.

The thirst to express myself in words can be severe, but for every word you see in these pages there are a dozen hesitations, fumblings and false starts. Content is the great beast when you are writing something as ambitious as a full-length book rather than, say, a wine review or a haiku. Seeing that the book is about me, based on my Parkinson's experiences and my reactions, I cannot simply get onto the Internet and look my material up. I need to outline, chop and dice themes and sub-themes, but also come into communication with the Parkinson's-beset body and brain. When I feel a trembling in my hand or in my leg, when I experience my back arching, my body sagging, I sometimes open into verdant verbiage. I have a feeling that the Parkinson's disease, the medication, or both are agitating my cognitive faculties. There is possibility in this for a word juggler. The brain effect does not have to be bad, at least until it all shuts off for good.

*When you face great challenge, and the usual
tools fail, you can always navigate by the stars.*

Athena Watches

Athena is out there to give men courage, and she approves of this message.

Strange to think, at this point in my life, I persist in the opinion that men and women differ. I should have a more thorough understanding of men than I do of women. I have, after all, logged considerable experience (that is pronounced "trial and error") as a man. I have had wives—yes, plural—and a son. I have had a business. I have both owed money (though not at present), and have had the onerous task of collecting it from others (some of whom, theoretically, still owe it from long ago—*you know who you are*).

I have never been a soldier, but I know that all maleness involves some kind of soldiering: the tasks soldiers *usually* do, surviving, getting rained on, enduring mud and slime, peeling potatoes, hauling out the trash. Glory is extremely rare in life, and then, *Sic transit gloria mundi*: when it comes, it leaves. You cannot count on fine moments. Everyday life is the vein you must mine. It is one of those mines from a western, with grimy desperadoes out there waiting to steal your gold. If you finally do get down the mountain to the assay office, people in suits rob you with a pen. You do what you can with what remains. Parkinson's disease like any malady presents the same issue: you do what you can with what remains.

Despite the wonderful quote from the song "Lola" by Ray Davies of the Kinks—"girls will be boys and boys will be girls/it's a mixed up muddled up shook up world"—I think the contrary applies: except for certain people who are genuinely confused, men are men and women are women. You hear popular talk of a man getting in touch with his "feminine side." Claptrap. Men do not have feminine sides. Oh, they do have receptive abilities, nurturing instincts, gentle and sensitive aspects, but they are receptive, nurturing, gentle or sensitive as men, not as women. These sides of the male persona are admirable—necessary—just as strength, perseverance, courage and the like are indispensable in their female manifestations. Male nurturing and female nurturing, male courage and female courage, are not identical. I can sense and even gape in awe at these qualities in a woman, but I can go further than that and live them as a man. My Parkinson's struggle is that of a man, and I cannot escape that. My challenges stand before me. If I try to run from them, they only loom larger.

The fact that the female is outside our male cognizance presents us with a great trap when we forget the fact that women, individually and in general, are real, not our fantasies. (I cannot speak of the distortions women may make of men in their imaginations, but undoubtedly I have female counterparts who may treat this issue.) It is useful to look into distant mythology to find meaning that rings true in the here and now. One man, who represents the blundering all of us undergo from time to time (or in perpetuity, in the case of those of us who really *are* fools) was Paris, prince of the royal house of Troy. Troy is in ruins now, buried beneath successor cities that are themselves buried, all the fault of Paris.

Eris, the goddess Discord—nasty, for sure—threw the apple of discord among the gods. Picture this sphere as about as benevolent as a hand grenade. On it was engraved the rubric "for the fairest." Zeus, king of the gods, lacked the confidence to tackle the question of who among the goddesses qualified. Zeus was no slouch, however. He had a W.C. Fieldsian instinct for finding a sucker. Paris was a natural.

Paris chose Aphrodite as "the fairest," spurning the goddesses Hera and Athena, because Aphrodite promised him the most beautiful woman in the world, Helen, whom Paris had to abduct to get, causing a war of revenge, devastation, and ruin. This war was a cauldron that tested the mettle of every one of its participants, Trojan or Greek. The twin epics it spawned, Homer's *Iliad* and *Odyssey*, raised questions relating to the male role that we have been debating ever since. It is well that women today demand equal time, but when you look at epics—Achilles, Odysseus, Aeneas, Beowulf, Roland—the arc of the story is male. If you are a woman writer, you might take this cue to create the great female epic. My brain is male, and I would be unable to touch this story from the inside.

Put me in the place of Paris. The result will be different. I am glad of Aphrodite, but I am not calling her to my corner. Aphrodite is called the "goddess of love," but she is better termed the goddess of the "narrow feminine archetype," that fantasy woman every man wants but who will never be. Fantasies are about as fleeting as glory, even if they appear more often. Fantasies do not work. They are fun when we perceive them as fun, ruinous when we confuse them with reality. Aphrodite does not understand Parkinson's. She lacks the perspective.

From what I know of Hera, wife of Zeus, I would have to be alone on a desert island to have anything to do with her, you would have to hold a gun to my head, I would have to be sure it was loaded and that you would actually pull the trigger. I have run across Hera many times in my transit across the arc of life. I have paid my dues. I am already on her bad side, so these words should not make my lot on this earth any worse. Hera does not understand Parkinson's. She is too proud to grasp the fragility disease can bring to a man.

I will take real women in the real world as they present
themselves, without expecting of them the benefits and
burdens of a goddess, but if I must have an archetype, let it
be Athena, so-called goddess of wisdom, though I would
rather call her "goddess of considering the moral basis of
action." When Jason set sail in his ship, the Argo, in search
of the golden fleece, Athena guided the crew through the
greatest of perils. When spiteful Hera sent Hercules on his
mighty labors, Athena stood beside him and allowed him to
prevail. Athena stood behind Theseus as he slew the
Minotaur. Athena guided Perseus in his high-risk raid on
the terrifying Gorgon Medusa. Athena protected Odysseus
during his ten-year ordeal after the sack of Troy. She
inspired his son Telemachus to seek his father and protect
his mother Penelope from the relentless suitors. Athena is
responsible for great things: the courage of action, to be
sure, but also the courage of endurance. For every morsel
of action, we live a thousand chunks of endurance. Athena
not only understands Parkinson's, she throws it as a
challenge at my feet. Soldier on, she exhorts. No excuses.
No whining. Victory can be yours.

Athena is a demanding goddess. She is both a war goddess
and the goddess of peaceful assembly and political affairs.
She protects the brave, in all aspects of life, but she does
not give them their bravery. Instead she expects it. Athena
sets the highest of standards.

Men have enough of their own momentum toward baser
things in life: appetites and all that. Athena provides a
balance: an austere standard of heroism, integrity,
intelligence, capability, leadership. Athena represents the
finest attributes women bring to the table of life. You can
get kissing and snuggling with a real woman, you can

certainly get nagging, but if you are talking about a goddess looking over your shoulder, Athena is the one who can really help you make the most of yourself. Athena is not your wife, not your girlfriend, not your sister, not your mother, not your beloved nanny, and yet she is a woman, that other phenomenon out there, that *difference*. One of your teachers—the one who first credited you with intelligence and judgment perhaps—may have been Athena. That wonderful real woman in your life takes on what you think is the beauty of Aphrodite not because she is Aphrodite but because she is Athena. *Athena* is the fairest.

You, reader, may actually be a woman. Good for you. Keep at it. You can see Paris for the dolt he really is. I do hope he is not *too* familiar to you. You are right to want your man to be a hero, to look to Athena for his standard, not a shoot-em-up action hero to be sure, but the do-the-right-thing workaday hero just the same. Everything a man does well—be it leading, be it nurturing—he does with courage. Do not think for a moment that this courage is bluster, bravado, or boast. It is difficult, multi-dimensional, and exacting. Men do not understand their courage, yet they have no choice but to live it. Athena stands and reminds them.

I have previously stressed that I am a non-believer. What I write about Athena is consistent with that statement. I do not "believe" in Athena, or any of the other Greek and Roman gods, as the ancients undoubtedly did. They are nevertheless with me as part of the culture I revere, as archetypes, swirling in my head. They stand on call during the good days, come to my aid or even challenge me on the trying days, ever at the ready as I walk my rocky road.

*In a Parkinson's world, a shower can easily turn
into a slippery mess of blood and soap.*

Cleaning Myself

The trick is to attend to the parts, hoping they add up to a cohesive whole.

Before Parkinson's disease, I would brush my teeth, shave, shower, and go out into the world without giving these processes much thought. That was, alas, before. The before is now ended. The Parkinson's now has its own peculiarities and strictures. The now turns what should be everyday actions into special events, habitual tasks into achievements. The big problem with these achievements as they pertain to keeping myself clean is that all the effort is only good for a single day. Come tomorrow, I will have to break through the barrier all over again.

My impaired sense of balance and my inability to coordinate body systems mean that I cannot simply accomplish a muscular movement, I must rather will it, solidify that will, and then grind my way through it. Fortunately, my thinking brain still works well, allowing me to construct and follow a mental checklist for each critical self-cleaning process. Without being so determinedly proactive, I would be lost, unshaven, half-clean, sweaty and miserable. The effort comes at a price however: fatigue, the necessity to recover and regroup.

Shaving usually comes first. Each morning as I rise, I feel an insistent need to get the hair off my face as soon as I can, as if it besmirches me. Since I am profoundly right-handed, I need to squirt the shaving foam into my left palm, even though my left ring and pinky fingers often vibrate from the Parkinson's. I lack the confidence to apply the foam to my face with the left hand, however, and so I transfer the foam to my right palm, as efficiently as possible. The Parkinson's sometimes makes my jaw pulsate, often precisely while I am oozing the foam across my chin. The pulsating deadens sensation across my jaw and face, so I really do not get the feeling I have applied the foam properly, even though the mirror tells me I have.

Standing at a sink, my body sways backwards and forwards, side to side. I keep a hand towel hanging from a hook to my left side. I grasp the towel with my left hand to steady myself as I methodically shave off the foam using my right hand. Since I am invariably in my socks, it helps my balance to stand on a plush bath mat. I need to use both hands to rinse off my face over the sink, but here the bending over position enhances the balance. As I dry my face using both hands, I depend on the rubbing motion to keep my body aligned. Nicely cleaned of stubble, I enjoy caressing my cleanly shaven face with my right fingers and palm, even as the left hand shakes. I have successfully shaved, and now the twenty-four hour clock starts ticking off the time before I will have to do it all over again.

For me to wash my full body, I need to follow a carefully constructed plan. There is no such thing in my world as simply hopping into the shower. Balance is the key issue, but there is also the question of coordination. I start by shampooing (what is left of) my hair. I try to cup my left fingers to squirt on shampoo, but the Parkinson's trembling makes it difficult for me to keep the fingers from gapping, and often shampoo will seep to the floor to foam up at my feet. Although my left arm is weak, I am able to carry the shampoo with it for a top-of-head deposit before engaging my right hand to suds it all around. I feel as if the stream of water cascading from the showerhead is providing me with a mooring instead of beating me down. Once I suds up, I need to do some challenging balance and pivot work to remove the shampoo and moisten the rest of my body for effective soap application. I know I waste water, but my inability to sense soap on my scalp leads me to rinse again and again, just in case. I over-rinse every other body part for the same reason. I have problems feeling clean so I have to engage my cerebellum to attain a state in which I know I am clean beyond doubt—and then move to the next hurdle.

With Parkinson's I do not fully feel many of the body movements I used to take for granted. I know, for example, that I soap under my left arm using my strong right hand, but I need to do this at least twice for me to feel wholly clean in the underarm region since my body does not give me good feedback. I have the opposite problem trying to soap my right underarm with my left hand: I feel the reception of the action on the active right side but remain uncertain as to the doing of the action with my compromised left hand and arm. Two soapings are a minimum. I soap up the center of my front torso using my right hand, but I need here to realign my balance constantly. I switch back to difficult left hand action to get the right edges of my torso, and strain to extend the washcloth to cover some of my back. To get the back itself, I switch back to a right hand approach and slide the soapy cloth down my back, letting go and catching it with my left hand. Here I count on the friction of the cloth on my back to give me enough time to switch hands. If the cloth falls to the bottom of the tub, I risk falling when I attempt to retrieve it.

Every time I complete a body area, I slather on a layer of fatigue along with the soap, but there is nowhere to rest and recharge in a shower. My next step is to get my rump, thighs and legs, with each availing myself of the sliding quality of the soapy cloth in contrast to its friction. I need to balance on one foot to get the other. This is always tenuous. When switching feet I need to compose myself a moment, align myself, catch my breath. I am a land creature, un-fond of water. I know I am reaching a progress point when the soaping is complete and the rinsing begins. If I do not like water, I like the soaped feeling less. Raising either arm, especially the left, is difficult for me. Positioning my underarms under the static shower stream requires contortion. I need to pirouette under the shower blast to assure a complete rinse, a maneuver I would find difficult even with shoes, much less in an aqueous soap-filled, steam-rich milieu.

I feel a wave of fatigue and balance interruption as I turn off the water. My aching need is to get a towel around my head, since my head hates wetness most of all. Leaving the bathtub is the most dangerous part of the process. I have never fallen in the shower but have twice lost my balance just outside the tub and careened back in butt first. To prevent this, I keep my thick bath mat perpendicular to the tub so with a single movement I can exit the tub and get my back to the wall rather than the tub. If I fell backwards here the wall would catch me. As in washing and soaping myself, I have more trouble drying my right side with my tenuous left hand than drying my left side with my good right hand. The left fatigues almost instantly, nor can it feel a towel's progress well. I get most of my body well dabbed, but I lack the coordinating strength to rub the wetness off completely—for my final step, I air-dry reclining on a towel on my bed. The air-drying is a rest and regeneration segment for me. A moment does come when I feel fully dry, fully rested, and fully clean. As with the shaving, of course, that twenty-four hour timer starts to tick. I hate water so much that even if I sweat up later, a second shower the same day is out of the question.

For my dental routine, I must move the plush mat from its position perpendicular to the back of the tub to the front of the sink. This prevents the door of the bathroom from closing. I push the door back until the edge of the bathtub buttresses it, lean back on the door for my own support, and carefully floss my teeth. The back and forth shaking of the flossing compromises my balance totally, and so I must lean back onto a surface. Once I have flossed my teeth and rinsed out the particles, I move onto the mat and lean over the sink to electric brush my teeth. Every time I adjust the direction of the toothbrush, I need to rebalance. For some reason, the towel I use to support myself while I am shaving does not work well while I am brushing my teeth, so instead with two left fingers I probe into the little overflow holes at the edge of the sink for stability. I brush the teeth one quadrant at a time, but my back usually gives in about three-quarters of the way through. I straighten up a moment, try to crack my back, and then bravely carry on.

As I am not in the habit of paying for manicures and pedicures, my final ablutionary torture involves paring my fingernails and toenails. My advantage here is that I can sit down. The fingernails go fairly smoothly, although I need to really concentrate when I use my non-dominant left hand to clip the right nails. If my left hand trembles, I need to wait out the shakes. Scrunching over to cut my toenails takes concentration and purpose, and usually a rest after each toe to catch my breath. I get the job done, but often have no choice but to reward myself with a substantial lie down. Clean, finally, but at a price, and the nails are only going to grow back.

*

When I wash my face at my bathroom sink, I usually take a good look at it to see what it is telling me. I wait with patience, but I get very little back.

166

The Parkinson's face is so often stone, but there is beauty in stone.

Stone Face

My brain tells my face to react, but the face refuses to obey.

I feel paroxysms of personality straining within me, but, when I face another human, he or she sees only an impenetrable stone face. French neurologist Jean-Martin Charcot, who coined the term "Parkinson's disease" long after Parkinson's death, added the stone face symptom to Parkinson's original list, writing that, "the muscles of the face are motionless, there is a remarkable fixity of look, and the features present a permanent expression of mournfulness, sometimes of stolid-ness and stupidity."

Just as Parkinson's has flattened my voice, the disease has short-circuited the ability of my face to express emotion, to light up with joy, to express frustration, and, especially, to smile. My face is impassive as if it were not even made of flesh. Like most human faces, mine has at least forty-three muscles. In my brain, the neurotransmitter dopamine, which controls muscles, has difficulty sending commands to those facial muscles. As a result, like many Parkinson's patients, because of my unmoving face I often seem uninterested in conversational topics, bored, or downright catatonic when in reality the personality behind my face is motivated to learn as much about other people as possible. I react inside to what other people are saying or projecting, but the reaction rarely shows on my face (or for that matter in non-verbal gestures, like arm movements). Having this stone face is a curse. I can assure you, it is not me. I am not the Parkinson's mask I unwillingly wear. I feel much emotion, even joy, inside, it just has difficulty coming out.

I began to notice my expressionless face a few years before the onset of the physical problems, like hand trembling and balance issues, that would eventually lead to my Parkinson's diagnosis. On one particular occasion a few years before the physical problems became clear, I visited my language club for dinner, sat at the French table, and got a chiding from several ladies about my tendency not to smile. One, someone I fancied, teased me mercilessly, begging me with clasped hands to smile like everybody else. My French works best when I am calm, and, being flustered, I lost speech entirely, retreating into a meal that I was not able to enjoy. I finally answered, in English, that I did not know how to say that smiling was overrated *en français*, but I did not truly believe it. I knew something was wrong with me. I looked around the table and at the other tables for different languages—Spanish, German, Italian—and noted how physically animated many of the people were. The operative phrase was joy at communicating. I yearned to radiate joy myself. Why was this path closed to me? My self-explanation at the time was my unfortunate brain wiring, reaching back to the silence I endured in early childhood. I have no way to prove it now, but I tend to suspect the problem was dopamine-related, a foretoken of the full-blown disease.

"How soon my sorrow hath destroyed my face," laments King Richard II in the Shakespeare play. When I think of that immortal line, I fear for my own compromised face. And to think that I slather moisturizing cream on it every night. What for, if the machine is broken on the inside? I identify with poor tragic Richard, hounded and ousted from his rightful throne as anointed king. I wish for no kingdom or throne, but I do so want the dignity of my face back.

Another incident, which occurred about six months before my emergency room visit, rings particularly strongly. I was out in Albuquerque with a lady-friend. I had one thing on my mind, but she had something else on her mind and since the woman is always right we were out on Rio Grande Boulevard at a rock club, and boy was it loud. Talk about sensory overload. The band was good solid roots rock. I wished I could sit in with my guitar, but I felt abidingly old compared with most of the crowd. Across from where we sat, we noted a black man in a suit. You do not see many black people in Albuquerque, and in that crowded bar, he was the only man in a suit. He sipped beer demurely. We determined that it was likely that he was a cop, and, in fact, a few days later the police shut the place down. No one could figure out why, but the whisper was major drug trafficking. The man looked our way, walked over to us, and told me he had never seen anyone who looked so "serious." I did not know what to say, forced a smile, shrugged off the remark, but I knew he was on to something. For a moment, I ascribed my demeanor to the pulsating noise and all the people, but I realize now that, even then, I knew something was not firing properly in my brain. In the back of that brain, not knowing anything about Parkinson's disease, my calculations involved aging, dementia, Alzheimer's, teenage drug use, Asperger's syndrome, and a range of complex emotional and psychological issues. A person's face is his window on the world. Mine hid behind curtains and shutters, closing me off, gagging me. The incident still frightens me, but at least the cop did not arrest me for criminal catatonia.

The way I look at other people often gives me trouble. Unmitigated by the distraction of facial signals, my stare cuts, and my hazel eyes are piercing. A few times a year I will be introduced to someone, invariably a woman, in a social situation, and she will recoil from my eyes, demanding, "Why are you looking at me like that?" If I stare—I know it is rude—I do not intend to. Looking outward rather than into myself, I cannot observe the manner of looking that causes such consternation. The question, in fact, takes me by surprise in the same way that my odd look obviously takes the other person by surprise. Appropriate facial movements would perhaps mitigate the effect, but these do not fire up. I do not know how to answer the question. I demur, averting my eyes, giving the other person a chance to escape. It has come to my mind that instead, when it happens again, I should stress the fact that without a mirror I have no way of knowing what "looking at me like that" means, but that perhaps the look is the result of a neurological condition I endure, and can they be more specific? This ought to tend to continue rather than cut short the conversation. The hidden benefit of this tactic is that at my age many of my contemporaries also have health issues—in talking about mine we could move on to theirs. We could find a common thread, leading to a stimulating "organ recital." I always look for a positive aspect to my difficulties, and a good solid health conversation qualifies.

Look for something positive long enough, and you will find it. My impaired ability to express myself physically has two clearly positive aspects. Others have long remarked at my skill at deadpan humor. Wit plus stone face makes almost anything funny. That is an asset when you intend humor, an annoyance when you do not. The stone face is also handy when you are playing the game of poker. The problem with poker is the fact that, like life itself, you can look at your cards and find them downright terrifying. You can trade in some cards and draw others now and then, but the Parkinson's card is one you must play. If you look carefully, you can see my reaction to that card written, in stone, on my face.

*

The stone face, as we shall see, does me no help when I am sitting across a table from a potential relationship partner.

Dating is actually a scam perpetrated by the powerful deodorant and mouthwash lobbies.

Dating the Parkinson's Way

When they notice me trembling, do they think it's them?

I am a single gentleman. Although I did not put the pieces together until much later, one of the first times I sensed I had something neurologically wrong with me was on a blind date in month one of my illness and diagnosis sequence, a January. I was still living in Albuquerque, New Mexico when the incident occurred. This is germane because of the altitude there—the city is a mile high—and it was not unusual for me to feel a little light headed from time to time and blame it on the thinner air. I had been seeing a woman named Marcia who, because she had not yet gotten over her previous boyfriend José, had made it clear to me that we were to "see other people." I had been of a mind that I really could have had a relationship with Marcia, but, not one to argue (and being tired of hearing about José), I reluctantly started on match.com (again). The result was that I had a date to meet a woman named Tracy. I suggested Bravo's Italian restaurant in Albuquerque Uptown for wine at six pm. The place is nice and quiet. Just as I was about to leave my apartment for the restaurant to meet Tracy, Marcia called and suggested we have dinner that very night. I thought fast and suggested 7:30. Despite Marcia's insistence that we see other people, I was not about to volunteer that I was meeting another woman at six. The meeting times would just dovetail.

I was tense when I met Tracy. The chemistry was instant. The problem was, pre-wine, my head was bobbing along on the ceiling. My heart was beating rapidly. I was edgy and off balance. I ascribed this to a combination of Marcia-anxiety, time management, and the usual culprit, the altitude. I told Tracy I felt uncomfortable and weird, and that it was not her. Maybe the wine would help. It did not. Maybe I should pace around a bit. That did not work. An experienced blind-dater, I figured I could stay the course, but less than ten minutes into the date I had to leave most of my good Tempranillo unconsumed and excuse myself. This was the only time in my life that I have hurriedly dropped bills onto a table the way they do in the movies. Only later did I recognize that episode as Parkinson-related. I recovered in time to meet Marcia for dinner. A few days later Tracy and I met in Albuquerque Old Town and had a proper New Mexican lunch at the Church Street Cafe. Marcia soon ended our relationship and Tracy and I began ours. It had a beginning, a middle, and an end, but the head on the ceiling episode did not recur, although we chuckled about it. Yes, in case you wonder, I do change some names in this section.

Soon after the relationship with Tracy ended (why it ended is grist for a different mill), in mid-June, I was at an outdoor singles mixer in the Albuquerque foothills (about six thousand feet above sea level) when my left foot seemed to merge into the patio. I was in the middle of a conversation with a woman who presented possibilities when this happened. I tried walking around, but just could not regain the feeling in the foot. I took myself home early and took an Ambien to get to quick sleep. A week later I was trying to shave when the foot seemed to collapse under me, I felt the first episode of hand tingling, spent a useless fourteen hours in the emergency room, had days of severe leg pain, and could not breathe. In August, I moved back to New York, the location of most of my family, figuring I would get better medical care (I also missed my young nieces). I changed locations on my match.com profile and started New York dating in September of that first year of trouble. I would not be misdiagnosed with MS until May of the next year (month seventeen), and would not be properly diagnosed with Parkinson's until the January after that (month twenty-five), but I knew I had something wrong with me. A doctor led me to believe it was primarily an orthopedic problem: pounding pain in my left leg. The arm and hand problems seemed to subside for a time. Dating reoccupied my reveries.

That autumn I had dates that went nowhere with Jane, Lucy, Olga, Nadine, Lori, Francine, Terri, Martha and Pat. You need to run through a few to meet that special someone. I met gestalt psychotherapist Marianne on a cold late November day at Bistro 12 in Tarrytown, New York. Feeling immediate chemistry, we kissed over the table. We met again in Manhattan at the J.P. Morgan Library. It was while viewing the interesting Edgar Allen Poe exhibition that I had what I call an attack: a weak prickly feeling on my left side and extreme lack of confidence in my left leg combined with balance difficulties. I felt like lying down but there was nowhere to go. I got through the museum, however, and dinner afterward. We saw each other a third time, going to a party in Soho and then having dinner at Dos Caminos restaurant on Hudson Street where I introduced Marianne to Mezcal, but afterward neither of us called the other. Perhaps I should have held onto this one, but I still remembered the illness I had at the Morgan Library and I had a crisis of confidence. She lived deep in New Jersey, and I used this as an excuse, but I liked her. Still, I felt the relationship to be tainted by what I later was to realize was Parkinson's. I felt that as a psychotherapist she sensed it before I did. This is just imagination. This could have been a real romance.

My next date was Myra, whom I met in Grand Central Terminal. We simply sat at one of the tables in the food court without ordering anything. Myra was a real animal lover, and I am not. From the beginning, it was apparent that this was not going anywhere. I was unconsciously holding myself with Parkinson's stiffness. She remarked that it was obvious I was not feeling well. I agreed. She suggested physical therapy. I was still six months off from my first neurologist visit. After we parted company, I walked into cold Manhattan to attend a professional wine show up on Madison Avenue, looked but did not taste, and took the train home, shivering with both the cold and with undiagnosed Parkinson's disease. I took Myra's advice and did two months of physical therapy.

Laurie, Francesca, and Carolyn that winter were duds, I took three months off from dating, and the next March (month fifteen) arranged to meet Brenda (or was it Janet?), an artist, at the Landmarc restaurant in Time Warner Center. I got to the building a good half hour early. I felt awful trembling and paced around the lobby, up and down the stairs, to try to work it off. I must have been extra jittery by the time the woman joined me for lunch, but I know from public speaking experience that most nerves actually do not show (unless you let them). I think it was that moment when I became sure I had a neurological problem, not just a bad leg, but the prospects petrified me, and, besides, here was a woman, naturally tense, shaking my hand and forcing a smile. First things first—force my own smile and ask her about herself. The first thing to come out was her revelation that she was really seventy when her match.com profile said sixty-five. She showed me photos of her oil paintings. I approved, we lunched, we parted. I did not call her again, thinking at first it was because of her age-fraud. A lot of women sculpt years off their age on these online dating services, but often they fess up before they meet you. It sank in, however that the real reason I did not follow up with her was because her fraud highlighted my own—I had a serious health issue. I ought to disclose it even if my profile on match.com had my age and weight down accurately. Of course, it is impossible to disclose a malady when you do not know what you have. I met another artist, Alice, the next week for an interminable lunch at the Turkuaz restaurant at 100th Street and Broadway. Alice balked when I told her I admired De Kooning, Pollock and Rothko—not European enough for her. The conversation turned to the painfully stiff way I was holding myself. She urged me to get a diagnosis. I decided I would.

I also decided that I would not meet any further women until I found out what ailed me, but women kept getting in touch with me, and I kept uselessly meeting them. I met Liz, Eve, Jen, Colleen, Sloane, Melissa, Susan, and Lara that spring, Susan and Lara after my MS misdiagnosis. Sloane was an exceptional beauty, but the first thing she said to me was, "I just started smoking again so I could quit drinking." I then went on a dating hiatus for a solid nine months, feeling it was all hopeless, also feeling that now that I knew what I had (or so I thought), I needed to disclose it, not an easy thing to ask someone to buy into. A few months after my Parkinson's diagnosis I regained the confidence to re-join match.com. In my profile, after a good deal of insanely clever self-descriptive verbiage, I added an exculpatory paragraph: "I have a neurological condition that leaves me with a balance issue. It takes me a few moments to regain my balance when I stand up or sit down, or get into or out of a car. I deal with it. I am healthy underneath it all and do regular exercise." My thinking was that this disclosure got me off the hook. Women my age are more likely than not to have health issues themselves— high cholesterol, diabetes, osteoporosis, or who knows what—so my own health statement ought to encourage them.

Nancy, my first date after my re-emergence, seemed to be responding to me until she remarked on the discontinuity between the amusing things I was saying and the stiff impassive manner in which I held myself, especially my stone face. "Is that because of the neurological condition you wrote about in your profile?" "Yes," I answered, and told her what it was. That was that. It was just as well, since Nancy's online description of her body type as "average" was something of a stretch. Coats and sweaters were involved, yet I could swear Nancy was occupying two chairs. Fabric seemed to be exuding in all directions from the woman's indeterminate center. A few days later, I met Michele, a well-dressed, well-kept Italian woman who worked for a medical practice. I did not intend to, but we talked about my health. Lesley, Marion and Sue were cases of no chemistry, Cheryl was too recent a widow, Enid admitted she was still living with her "ex" husband, Robin grilled me like a steak, Reina was lovely, but I could not pin her down for a second date. I then moved into a period I started to call "Culture Alley." First, Sheila took five performing arts sorties to tell me she wanted nothing more, and then Carolyn took an even dozen strained expeditions to come to a similar pronouncement: four concerts, one play, four French films, and three art museums. (You are perhaps expecting a partridge in a pear tree.) Believe you me—my cultural enrichment was considerable.

There is more, stretching over an additional year, but I think you have had enough of this theme for now. I can tell, because I certainly have reached a saturation point with the subject. Let us just assume that the reason I do not click with any of these women is me, and not them, always me and never them. Even if we assume this, Parkinson's disease is something of a problem when it comes to these episodes. They see a face of stone, and hear a voice with little modulation. Oh, I hear the voice modulating expressively and feel the face reacting, but it does not transfer—the muscles do not get the signals I send them, the woman leaves the encounter with a blank, and the best I can do is add a positive note to the encounter by insisting on paying the check. This is uncharted territory for me, and I do not know what to do about it.

*

At the supermarket, my radar is up for eligible women—"Is that canned tuna really four for five dollars?"—If I force a smile, something might come of it, but smiles so often desert me, as I find shopping one of the grimmer and most debilitating of tasks.

Shopping

I know it's good for me—endorphins and all—but all the planning, card swiping, and being pleasant to clerks...

I was out on a blind date a few weeks ago with a woman who told me that one of her main passions in life was shopping. Buzz—next! I realize that shopping is important to the economy, but I find shopping for myself, particularly for clothing, extremely taxing. I need to admit that even before Parkinson's, shopping was very low on my priority list. Just as I was a reverse alcoholic, I was also a reverse shopaholic. I tended to avoid any form of retail therapy even though I knew that I could have used a few make-a-purchase endorphins. The online option works for me when it comes to clothing. Even if I persist in avoiding going physically shopping for clothing, I cannot avoid shopping altogether. Food shopping is a necessity. It is also invariably some kind of an ordeal.

Parkinson's gives me special problems when I need to push and navigate a shopping cart. Other people, many more agile than me, use the same space, and their actions and reactions can be unpredictable. I need to keep my radar going, keeping in mind that the disease diminishes my ability to judge distance and relative speed. I act as if I were inside a video game in which I must constantly deal with obstacles that pop up with lightning speed. Driving a car is easier than pushing a shopping cart because of the existence of lanes, stop signs and traffic lights. Besides, pushing an automobile accelerator requires less effort than shoving a steel cart, especially if you get one of the recalcitrant ones. I have become fairly good at stationing the cart in a strategic location and doing a foray on foot, a technique that is particularly effective in the anxious rows where the market displays dairy and meat. Avoiding other moving carts is a constant concern. I realize these carts are piloted by thinking humans like me, but I assume total distraction on their part. I have to do the avoiding, just to be on the safe side.

Filling my shopping cart presents me with challenges. As I teeter, it is no easy task for me to reach up for an item or bend down for an item, grab just one, lean over the cart and place the item into the cart without dropping it. When I accomplish this task, I am ever aware of the shopping cart traffic that buzzes ahead and behind me. When I stand up suddenly from a bend-down, I run the risk of getting a dizzying head-rush. Fortunately the cart itself acts as a mooring and it is easy to grab so I can ride out the feeling. If I find myself in a quiet aisle, I lean over the cart for ten or fifteen seconds to get my breath back after I need to do an oomph kind of movement. If the aisle is congested and I have no opportunity to rest, I try to get some rhythm out of the cart pushing. I have the option of shopping at two locations of my supermarket chain. I patronize the one farthest away from me because I like the layout better— anything to make the exhausting effort of filling that cart more efficient (the parking is also easier).

One of the most trying sections of the food shopping experience comes at the supermarket deli counter. I am on the spot. I must stand for a few minutes and avoid keeling over. Parkinson's gives me a soft voice, and I need to take special pains to project that voice when I give my order: "Pound of sliced ham and half pound coleslaw." The deli man is often kind enough to offer me a free slice, which means unfortunately that I must challenge my balance by bending over the large counter to accept the slice and push out a feeble "thank you," all at the same time. To avoid these transactions, the balancing and the waiting, I sometimes buy the pre-packaged deli, but it is never as good. Once the deli man hands me the carefully packaged items, I slip them into the cart and lean on it to get my bearings again. I make sure not to forget that final "thank you" and then press on to further fill the cart.

With the physical limitations of Parkinson's, it is more than a task to place items from a shopping cart onto the checkout belt. Of course I place my keys with my super-saver tag on the belt before all else. If I have many items, I have filled the main basket of the cart. I must get in front of the cart to reach in deep for my items, circling the cart when I finish with these items to get from the other direction the items I have placed in the convenient child seat area in front of the cart handle. I feel the backward pressure of the person ahead of me and the impatience of the people behind me. I consider how much effort it will take for me to extract my credit card, swipe it, sign my name if they ask me. Will they finish checking all the items while I am still fumbling for my wallet? They give you that aggrieved look if you slow them down. I do not feel obliged to smile at the checker and at the bagger, but I do, thanking them, never failing to remark to myself once I am finally free of this ordeal that my money is just as good without the smile. I am not getting any younger. Why scrunch my face unnecessarily? It is not as if I can go home and iron off the wrinkles.

At one specialty market I frequent (all right, forget the needless anonymity, it is Trader Joe's), the checkers do something truly inspired: they empty your cart for you (and they are energetically efficient). This practice is advanced, a true slice of gentle civilization in a world that is so very hard for a Parkinson's person. Their prices are fair as well. I cannot find everything I want at Trader's Joe's, but I rely on them for a lot of my staples, my almonds and sunflower seeds, and especially for the lack of hassle at the checkout. The freedom from the need to scan that little key tag is also something of a plus, removing one more transaction from the checkout process. When the clerks at Trader Joe's wish me a nice day, I get the notion that they mean it, and my smile is often the real thing. They seem to know me, they see me shuffle and struggle, and they help me. I can only be grateful.

Flowers are restful to look at. They have neither emotions nor conflicts.

—Sigmund Freud

My Emotional State

It depends on forging ahead, creating, refusing ever to stop.

You know you have a sidekick who is never going to go away. You hope, you fancy, you puff yourself up, but no amount of self-talk is going to push aside the basic fact that you have a chronic disease. Reality is an important concept, and not always as obvious as it should be. Without reality, you might as well spend your time choosing ancestors with legendary wealth, enduring health or both. Playing the lottery gives you at least a sliver of reality (and sometimes you do win four dollars), but wishing you did not have a disease does not. Run from reality and you run from yourself. Embrace reality and you prove you are not a fraud. You win a small victory. You look for other small victories—today was not such a horrible day—even if these victories are sandwiched in stark ignominious defeat: fatigue, stumbling, involuntary muscle movements, and no cure. Keeping to an even emotional keel in the face of Parkinson's disease is priority one, your mooring in a sea into which you could easily sink. To do this, you need purpose beyond the physical act of enduring.

Purpose, and the emotional stability it brings, lives in my mission as a writer. Writing redeems me. The word count at the lower left of my screen proves that I accomplish something. I am always open to the notion that some of it is gibberish, but I know that even the nonsense I sometimes write can function as the germ of some quality philosophizing (if I only work hard in revising it). In America, the land that I love, we live in an important cultural continuum that demands that one day or even each day we must account for ourselves. Going to bed with clean teeth is important. So is going to bed snuggled up with a messy basket of ideas. When morning comes, I can start mucking up the teeth again, and key in the ideas. I bask in the insistent glare of my word count.

Before you protest that my word count is mere quantity, let me defend myself by asserting that I only arrive at quantity by picking up the sponge of my being and wringing out quality. I admit I am prolific—novels, poems, essays, songs, guidebooks, a musical comedy—but I never take my penchant for output for granted. As soon as I have my morning tea, I place my unpadded butt in my seat and get to work. This is my everyday existence, and I find value in it, even though it filters through my Parkinson's brain. Is my strong self-image simply a given, a card dealt by destiny's hand, or have I built it over the decades out of pieces of my life? I look into these issues because it seems that I am less emotionally down than I think I ought to be, considering the Parkinson's disease. Am I feeling from the disease some kind of cerebral silver lining? Or is it the enhanced level of dopamine because of the drugs I take? Hope inflates me, despite the fact that I know there is presently no cure for what I have. That is for now. Those brain scientists are clever. James Parkinson wrote in his original 1817 essay that, "there appears to be sufficient reason for hoping that some remedial process may ere long be discovered, by which, at least, the progress of the disease may be stopped." I am not the only person with Parkinson's disease. Someone could make an awful lot of money figuring this one out. I not only want a heads up on the new drugs, I want to get in early on any related initial public offering.

If there is one down side to the notion that I enjoy positive brain chemicals it is the possibility that despite all my efforts the chemical balance could change for the worse. This is no good thought. I choose to believe that at least a kernel of my positive mood comes from inside me and has nothing to do with chemicals. If all I am is a chemistry set, why bother? Chemistry does not explain human subjectivity. My subjectivity is the notion that I am valuable (and I would add that I believe the entire human race is worthwhile). No objective standard for this belief exists—I must decide to believe, and stick with my decision. Brain chemicals might nurture the seed of hope inside me, but that hope is my creation, not theirs. I want to live some form of life, not some reverberation of Parkinson's disease. So far, I have succeeded in this. The artwork I now do might indeed be facilitated by the dopamine I swallow, but I am the artist, genuinely, honesty and with no excuse.

I feel a deep wholeness, an abiding one-ness, the sense that my seams are holding. So far…

When you appear to be one of the undead, you might as well make the most of it. Zombies are eternally popular.

Zombie

I feel a kinship with the army of the undead out there.

When I last visited my grandchildren in Australia, I thrust my arms in front of me and played zombie as they screamed in mock terror and delight. Even though I was jet-lagged and well fatigued, I discovered that the zombie act gave me some energy (although anything I do that will make a child squeal in delight ought to have the same effect). I developed lobsterman (menacing pincers made from toilet paper rolls) soon after, generating a good level of squeals, but not at the bloodcurdling level of the zombie reenactment. The success of my zombie has staggered through my brain in the several months since. I have begun to notice a number of television commercials that humorously feature zombies. Zombie references seem to abound. Just this morning on CNBC, they referred to zombie real estate. A zombie title occurs when a lender begins foreclosure proceedings on a property and then unexpectedly dismisses the foreclosure (it might not be worth the trouble), often without informing the occupant. If, relying on the foreclosure, the occupant moves out, he or she could unknowingly be liable for taxes, and maintenance and repairs. In 2011, the Centers for Disease Control published, *Preparedness 101: Zombie Apocalypse,* providing tips to survive a zombie invasion as a "fun new way of teaching the importance of emergency preparedness." There is even a cocktail called a zombie, made with several kinds of rum mixed with fruit juices. The idea is that after you consume the zombie, you will resemble one. If you have Parkinson's disease, you may well resemble one of the undead even before you order that cocktail.

Parkinson's disease freezes and stiffens me, making movement difficult and turning my face into an expressionless wasteland. In several key respects, the malady creates an army of zombies. I did not have to do military service during the Vietnam era because of the draft lottery, but I find myself conscripted into the zombie army today. I realize most passersby are completely neutral in their view of me, but I must occasionally pass zombie-phobes for whom my gait and my visage strike terror. In my own imaginings, I am terrified of the prospect of striking terror in others. I am a gentle, delicate man who hates to see squirrels run over in the street. You only have one chance at making a first impression. When someone likens you to a zombie, you are not getting off on the right foot. Most people do not think much about this, but, the highly paranoid aside, you expect to meet zombies only in your imagination. All of a sudden, here is the real thing, ready to make a meal out of human flesh. Your first impulse is not going to be to give that zombie a hug. Although you know in your mind that zombies are the stuff of fiction, in your heart lurks a seed of doubt. I am the victim of that doubt.

If I am not regaling my grandchildren, I do not wish to walk like a zombie, but the Parkinson's zombie master forces me. My upper body stiffens as the big torso muscles contract, stiffens still more as I try not to lean forward into my destination. I try to swing my arms like a normal non-zombie, but my arms have a strong tendency to hang limp and dead by my sides. I reach a true stride at some points, but a wave of fatigue short circuits the effort. I lurch forward spasmodically. I attempt to lift my feet and roll in my walk as suggested by my Parkinson's smart phone app but this only lends an additional artificial layer to my gait. I might be the first person to remark on the Parkinson's-Zombie connection, but it does seem so obvious to me that

I would be astonished if I were. Call us Parkin-bies. There are armies of us out there, ready to disrupt.

The people who pass me and make the zombie judgment will, it is true, pass elderly or disabled people, but while noting their challenges, will not make the zombie judgment as they do in my case. The elderly and disabled are essentially humans who try to move normally but who cannot do so because of some physical block. You can often see in their eyes that they are really trying. If you view one struggling to cross a street and are unable to assist, you at least become a rooter. Parkinson's locomotion is by contrast unnatural in its conception. You wonder why that odd person is not tapping into his obvious ability to walk like the rest of us. Why can't he simply decide to swing his arms—why can't he simply decide to stand up straight? It does not come to your mind that the person might have a problem with his brain that overrides his will. Without having a handle on the medical details, or even knowing that a medical issue is involved, you will have the natural tendency to dip into the popular imagination and arrive at a judgment of weird, strange, odd, and at some level chuckle to yourself: ah-ha, so this is a genuine zombie, something to tell the grandchildren.

My face is a zombie face, devoid of inflection, bereft of expression. The zombie face refuses even to register my struggle and frustration, projecting emotionlessly as if indistinguishable from the phalanx of the undead. The non-zombie expects the faces of others to register and interact and is offended when another human is too rude or self-obsessed to activate at least a cursory response. That rudeness, however, generally expresses itself on the face. Passing the Parkinson zombie, however, the non-zombie gets no reading at all. Humans are highly subjective, and do not expect to encounter objective-seeming automatons in human guise. Even when they cannot articulate why, they expect action from the human face, vibrancy, a sense that the other person is alive. Absent this subtle feedback, they make the subconscious decision that they are dealing with a zombie.

Moving from the face in general and focusing in on the eyes, I stare like a zombie. I stare into space and I stare at other people. My eyes glisten with involuntary tears. My eyes glaze over, as if the act of emitting cosmic rays from my dangerous eyes taxes them to the fullest. This condition often leads to the "Why are you looking at me like that?" response I have previously written about. I cannot very well answer, "Because I am a zombie," and so probably continue the stare as my brain whirrs excitedly in the distress this question always causes me. Implicit in the experience is the notion that my manner of staring at others is not quite human. Later, if they remember the incident and give me the benefit of the doubt they might, charitably in this case, decide that "Oh, he can't help it. He's a zombie after all. Look at him there, how his eyes glaze, how he stares into the distance, as if scanning the heavens for the saucer that will reunite him with his fellow zombie-aliens."

I speak with the voice of a zombie, listlessly, with scant vocal expression. My voice has lost the ability to modulate pitch and volume. I lack the breathing power to push out enough air to give my voice interest and inflection. My breathing itself is often just a thin, audible wheeze. Sometimes, when the Parkinson's saps me with fatigue, I also lack the will to verbalize. Because speech takes energy, I often sharply edit my speech, keeping to the necessary stitches and leaving out the embroidery. A nod will do when someone says hello. I show less verbal austerity when I write, but realize that I do this in manageable bits and am not subject to a real time clock. Put me in a real time vocalizing situation, wait just a few minutes, and watch the inner zombie take over. How many times have others signaled me—earth to Elliot? Before my zombie consciousness grew as the Parkinson's disease progressed, I used to use the term "catatonic" to describe the state in which I turned off when among others. This was getting close to the phenomenon, but not quite there. Catatonia applies to a human, while Parkinson's has caused me to lose touch with the essential human within me, as happens with any zombie.

Parkinson's disease is associated with slow movement and equally sluggish reactions. Does this remind you of zombies? I thought so. I put on and remove eyeglasses with deliberation. I am equally plodding when it comes to dressing and undressing, sitting down and getting up. As I have expressed many times in this book, the Parkinson's way of doing things is lurching, jarring, slow and discontinuous, very much the way a zombie operates. I decide on an action, do step one, step two, and so on, with zombie-like clumsiness rather than humanlike coordination. My inner life, my thoughts and feelings, are probably those areas in which I am least like a zombie. Although Parkinson's is an illness of the brain, it is not a malady of the mind. Deep within, my thoughts are quintessentially human, free and unfettered. Body and mind are on divergent paths, acting out different scripts. One special area in which I am far from a zombie is in sleep. My sleep is dream-filled, creative, luscious and fertile, a veritable garden of human wonder. I never seem to get enough. In sleep, I am human.

Parkinson's causes my body to tremble, especially my left side. My balance problem affects the whole body. I teeter both to the left and right and forward and backward. Visualize any typical assembly of zombies and you will note similarities: they tremble and quake, teeter and shake, whether they are milling about or moving forward in an organized mass to threaten the community. On my walks out there in my community, I feel most vulnerable when I have to stand still to wait at a pedestrian crossing. Wobbling and swaying, I imagine I am a zombie who has lost the protection of his group. I am only a moment away from generating mass hysteria. A few people look at me askance. A few more could form the nucleus of an enraged mob. Pitchforks might suddenly appear as they hunt me down and drive me out of town. Save me, oh green crossing signal. No one claims that the life of a zombie is easy! Everyone is out to get you when you are a zombie.

You live among others, but you can only live your own life.

Alone

It is all up to me.

I am a crossword puzzle junkie. Certain answers, usually short words, recur when you do puzzles frequently. "Alone" is one of those answers. The clue is "Admiral Byrd book." In 1934, Admiral Richard E. Byrd, who had already achieved fame for his flights over both north and south poles, attempted to spend six months near the South Pole, completely alone, "to taste peace and quiet long enough to know how good they really are." The expedition went badly for Byrd, both mentally and physically. The book *Alone* is a wrenching narrative of Byrd's struggle to survive. It became a national best-seller in 1938. The title—in fact the concept and the content—means a great deal to me. I have never felt more out of touch with the world around me as I have since my Parkinson's diagnosis. I could have entitled this book *Alone*.

The word "alone" applies to my own struggle to survive. Five simple letters distill my vexations, my uncertainties, my worry and even my hope. Other people suffer from Parkinson's disease, but no one else can bear *my* Parkinson's disease, my brain this time. The fact that Parkinson's is not one of those rare diseases is of no consolation to me. I feel still the rarity of this disease, in fact any disease, as a function of my own life. I have had my ailments and complaints over the years, but this is my first full-fledged disease. I have also had my periods of poor physical conditioning, being out of shape, but the several years before my Parkinson's downslide were among my most active—my passionate activity had been mountain hiking. Parkinson's came and wrenched me away from my beloved mountain. I did get some functionality back once I was properly diagnosed and medicated, but the top of that mountain seems truly a long way off.

The Buddha tells us, "No one saves us but ourselves. No one can and no one may. We ourselves must walk the path." Now, Buddha, I understand the truth in your statement, I alone must live my life. The problem arises when you consider that no matter how honestly and directly I live my life, the one thing I cannot cure on my own is loneliness itself. Another person is necessary to cure solitude. In the struggle for my life, can another person save me? The answer is no, but another person can certainly help me. I have no one. I am alone. Despite the fact that women can be maddening, and draining, I could surely use a helpmate now. I do not mean someone to lean on or to complain to, but rather someone to share experiences, to gnaw at life with me. My three sisters love me and provide a network for me, but they have their own lives and concerns, and I need more. I do not expect more from anyone at this time, and so I need to be my own helpmate, take my own counsel. I succeed in buoying myself often, but not always. Sometimes, treading water all too long, I feel I will sink. I am not expecting somebody to rescue me—I just want somebody to hold my hand now and then. I do not even have that. I am alone.

As a writer, assuming I do get a readership, even then the other people absorb my work product at their own pace, on their own terms, in their real time and not mine. I may touch an unseen audience now as I enter text, but the action is one-way, the colloquy entirely in my mind. Mario Vargas Llosa wrote, "Writing a book is a very lonely business. You are totally cut off from the rest of the world, submerged in your obsessions and memories." Tell me about it. I am writing about myself this time, even as I write for others, in the sputtering fancy that some of my readers will be able to relate to my words. My choice to work as a writer cuts me off from the rest of the world, dependent on my own subjectivity, rolling the dice in the gambler's hope that I will reach others, that my insights are interesting. Llosa fails to get into the issue of whether *his* obsessions and memories strike chords with the rest of humanity—we know that they do just as we know that mine might not get anywhere. I write…alone…with no guarantee that I will attain the immortality of language. All this effort, all these words, might vaporize into oblivion.

I was recently lying on my couch on a hot sticky June day, thinking nap, but I felt restless. An abiding sense of self-responsibility welled within me and forced me to slather additional emotion onto this screen. As I did, I felt a true pang of solitude, the whirling, menacing Antarctic snows of Admiral Byrd, the trepidation that you, yourself, will not be enough, even for yourself alone, the certainty that though death is indeed terrible, being forgotten is shades worse. A man wants in the minimum to be able to help himself, create an image that at least he will admire, and hope that others will see some of his self-construction as worthwhile. Even those writers who succeed in reaching others—and Llosa won the Nobel Prize—tread the lonely boards of the writing process with the knowledge that they strive to create in the shadow of failure, and completely alone. The muse may flee at any time. If I could snuggle up to my paragraphs and hug my sentences, I would, but they are not helpmates, they are hard taskmasters and leave me spent and alone.

According to Mark Twain, "The worst loneliness is not to be comfortable with yourself." I admit that this phrase strikes me hard. If I look into myself, I am deeply dissatisfied, tangibly uncomfortable, ill at ease, reluctant to sit down and have a talk with myself. Oh, I know I am interesting, others note this trait often enough, but I am not sure I am a person of quality, and by that I mean humanity. I am not comfortable with myself, not physically, not morally. Those three silent years at the start of my life left me with impossible heroic standards. I *am* clever, but I am also clever enough to see that cleverness for what it is: a deception and a crutch. I lean on my intellect to fill screen space just as I used to lean on lampposts to prevent myself from falling down into the street in a Parkinson's stupor. The writing process for me is no less comfortable than the physical strain I endure getting through a Parkinson's day. I suffer Twain's worst loneliness because I fear I am a fraud, a snake oil salesman, a dealer in smoke and mirrors, too clever for my own good. You probably want to talk me out of that view, but I am devious at self-damage, so do not even try.

I am not going to repudiate or delete the previous paragraph, but do project it as only one segment of my personality, which is complex. Yes, I am hard on myself and uncomfortable with myself, and I feel utterly alone. Of course, I know I am not a fraud, I just engage the self-critic a little too often and with a little too much acid. I have written about my fear of not being able to express myself, about being silenced. I tend to silence myself by claiming to myself that I am a fraud, relying on my cleverness, when I know there is more to me than that. Silence is the cousin of solitude. I am not comfortable with myself, but the discomfort has several dimensions. Half the time I am not comfortable with myself, and hence alone, because I doubt myself. The other half of the time, I am not comfortable with myself, and hence alone, because I do not believe in the crutch of comfort. Comfort dulls the edge of excellence. Creativity requires the discomfort of risk, when the heart beats sporadically and the stomach churns insistently. If being alone is the price for getting words onto a screen and giving them value, I will pay that price. The irony remains that I am alone if I create, and I am most alone if I do not create.

Mother Teresa remarked, "Loneliness is the most terrible poverty." This is perhaps true, but ironically did not Mother Teresa herself embrace a life of poverty? It is not necessary, you see, to enjoy this life of poverty to gain a benefit from it. Being alone is a process, not an end. Victor Hugo in *Les Misérables* writes, "It is nothing to die. It is frightful not to live." Much of this thing we call life is lonely. It is hence frightful not to be lonely, if in avoiding solitude one avoids the center of life. The Buddha states, "As you walk and eat and travel, be where you are. Otherwise you will miss most of your life." I have written already that I have difficulty reaching a state of flow, a condition of there-ness, but perhaps this is nothing but embracing the value of solitude, otherwise I miss most of my life. I can accept being alone, but that does not mean I do not feel pain. If life is pain, it is still more valuable than oblivion. If I exist, alone, I am at least one. After I am gone, subtract even that one. In the face of this, I will hold on to alone.

Endurance speaks its own language.

I Will Endure

It is the only choice.

When I first planned this final section, which I designed to be uplifting, I entitled it, "I Will Get Through All This." I soon realized that the title was inaccurate, however. I will not get through all this. James Parkinson wrote of the malady, "…the unhappy sufferer has considered it as an evil, from the domination of which he has no prospect of escape." There is no other side. Parkinson's disease has no cure. It is a one-way street. I might stabilize, things might get much worse, but, at best, I have Parkinson's for my allotment. What I can do is refuse to allow the disease to win. That is a realistic possibility. To reach that goal I need to reach deep into my being. Visualize a handful of glop. Insides are not pretty. I have written a story of myself that, while often amusing or stimulating, is, when you burn off the fat, hard and essentially grim. To win this game, I need to discover a glimmer of light. I need to endure. To do this, I will take a backward look at a pair of episodes in my life when I made the conscious decision to endure. I chose life then as I choose life now. I am powerful for having lived in the world. Nothing can stop me. I will endure.

The first incident involved a blizzard. In May of 1977 when my son was just two, we were alone together in my family's country house. The skies darkened and a few odd flakes of snow began to fall. We got excited at the prospect of maybe getting a touch of winter in the full of spring. But the snow kept coming, quickening its pace. People in the area still remember the unusual spring storm. Nature kept at it. The house lost power. I loaded us into the car, drove about a mile and a half down the mountain, only to have the car conk out in snowdrifts. We were not properly dressed for the weather. My only choice was to cradle my young son in my arms and trudge back up the hill to the house, blinding snow and wind driving into my face, my little boy convulsed in fearful tears, shivering and trembling. The trek back took more than an hour. I held him tight and put one foot in front of the other. The boy became heavier the longer I held him, but I could not put him down even for a moment. I might have stopped very briefly a time or two just to gather myself, but I did get him back into the house, we lit a fire, and all was well. Decades later, he does not remember, but I will never forget that time I endured. Elemental nature speaks with an insistent voice. When you are out in it, and you survive, you never forget the lesson.

Twenty-three years later, also in my birth month of May, in 2000, an episode occurred that put me a handshake away from death. I can still taste the cinders of death in the back of my throat. I had for years suffered from queasiness and faintness while having blood taken for tests. Through my twenties and into my thirties I got through this limitation by insisting on lying down while they took my blood. Thirty seconds after the nurse finished taking my blood, I could rise onto my feet without swooning. As I grew older, the problem seemed to diminish. I tried having my blood taken while simply sitting, I had no adverse consequences, and stopped making a fuss over the entire matter. I eventually got to the point where I felt I could donate blood. I recognized that for a donation they would take more blood than they would for a test, but I felt I should do my civic duty. I volunteered for a local blood drive. In a church basement, it was all going all right at first, then I felt a little queasy, and then suddenly my world went black. On the outside, the techs had put me on the floor, my breathing was zero, my pulse not measurable, my blood pressure non-existent. On the inside, I stood at a precipice, balancing on a ledge, feeling the brain activity of a thousand simultaneous dreams. The beyond beckoned, it seemed painless and sweet, I hovered a few moments but then clearly stepped back into reality. When I opened my eyes, I got the keen sense that I had chosen to endure, chosen life over death. I began to laugh, to the consternation of the extremely worried people who hovered around me. I could have jumped in and gone along with death. The techs administering the blood drive had no defibrillator or other lifesaving equipment. Maybe I would have come back from what they later termed a vasovagal reaction in any case (not everybody does), but I at least had the strong perception that I had actually decided to live. If you consider that I was on that date literally born again, I am barely out of my teens now. No wonder my face still breaks out.

Call me a born-again teenager, or call me middle aged, I today face a crisis much worse than a snowstorm or a medical wrong turn. I decide to live now, a life that is not only theoretical—the state of not being dead—but a life of quality and focus in the face of a major health issue. I decide not to cede to the blizzard. I shall not willingly cross the divide into the blackness. Ill health can be seductive. It deflates the requirement to achieve. The story is over already, so I will just go with the flow. I have had my life and now it has ended. We know that does not work. We have no choice but to live. Yet death, the antithesis of endurance, does seduce. This is because it is a liar. Death is anti-being, nothing, and yet we give it a personality. It is in our nature to personalize concepts. Embracing death accomplishes nothing. Life is all we have. Perhaps if I had a difficult cancer, I would refuse treatment like my cousin Peter did and accept my fate, but when the illness is chronic, and does not kill you readily, all giving in does is ensure a diminished life. There is no glory in such misery. My integrity gives me no choice but to endure. Furthermore, although most readers of this book will agree with my assessment of myself as pessimistic, at the base of it I believe in life for myself and for other people. I still have faith in the human race and its goodness. It stands to reason that I should include myself in that belief. *We* will endure.

If you have read this far, you must be praised for enduring the sorry catalog of my frailties, weaknesses and failings. The vast majority of people with Parkinson's disease, or, for that matter, with any serious disease, do not wallow in the muck of such detail. In my imagination lives an ideal Parkinson's sufferer who is better than me, who takes the malady and other life annoyances in his stride, uncomplaining, getting on with his life and career without a tenth of the thought about the disease as I give it. So be it. Such a Mr. Parkinson Perfect would probably think it an idle effort to commit all these thoughts and observations to text. So be it. He should not be too quick to criticize. He survives by bypassing the illness while I survive by subjecting it to the glare of introspection. He weaves his way through and around the illness while I try to chop it into little bits and spit it out. I am not likely to win by choosing this tactic, but I have no choice. My words represent my survival, my escape from inevitable pain.

Allow me to stress the word *my*. It is my brain this time. Does my stress on myself show that I lack empathy and compassion? I do not think so. I am leaving my inner self, all my trepidations and anxieties, open for all to see. I hope also that I have done so skillfully. I express my illness, my movement issues, my trembling, my stone face, with the hope that by some miracle these words will leap out of their medium and slither into the brains of others. I imagine another Parkinson's sufferer—not the perfect one—reading my words and nodding grimly, or getting a chuckle out of some other of my words—Yes, that is the way it happens to me! I work, I endure for just this prospect, for this mission, to see this book reach others and diffuse its way into the world of thought.

I also endure for the sake of people who love me, even—I am getting all too hopeful here—for people who simply like me. I have two cousins who have lost sons. They want me to endure. My three sisters want me to endure. My nieces and nephew want me to endure. My son and my three grandchildren want me to endure and even, if possible, enjoy myself over the years that remain. I certainly could not face any of these people, or any of my friends, and tell them that I have surrendered to Parkinson's disease. I do not expect any of these people to give in to life's cruel extortion. I would be a hypocrite if I did not myself live up to the standards I set for others. They will endure. I will endure.

About The Author

Wine and spirits educator Elliot Essman is author of the book *Use Wine to Make Sense of the World*. A native New Yorker, Elliot holds both Certified Specialist of Wine (CSW) and Certified Specialist of Spirits (CSS) designations from the Society of Wine Educators as well as a Wine and Spirits Educational Trust (WSET) Level 3 certificate. Elliot earned a James Beard Foundation Journalism Award nomination for his newspaper writing in the beer, wine and spirits category.

Dedication

To WLSC who taught me that it requires imagination to face up to the unimaginable.

9 798590 460601